# Springer Series
# on Geriatric Nursing

**Mathy D. Mezey, RN, EdD, FAAN, Series Editor**
*New York University Division of Nursing*

**Advisory Board:** Margaret Dimond, PhD, RN, FAAN; Steven H. Ferris, PhD; Terry Fulmer, PhD, RN, FAAN; Linda Kaiser, PhD, RN, ACSW; Virgene Kayser-Jones, PhD, RN, FAAN; Eugenia Siegler, MD; Neville Strumpf, PhD, RN, FAAN; May Wykle, PhD, RN, FAAN; Mary Walker, PhD, RN, FAAN

**Mathy Doval Mezey, RN, EdD, FAAN,** received her baccalaureate, masters, and doctoral degrees from Teacher's College, Columbia University. She taught at Lehman College in New York City and in the School of Nursing at the University of Pennsylvania, where she was Director of the Geriatric Nurse Practitioner Program. She is the past Director of the Robert Wood Johnson Foundation Teaching Nursing Home Program. Currently, she is the Independence Foundation Professor of Nursing Education in the Division of Nursing at New York University.

**Louise Hartnett Rauckhorst, RNC, ANP, EdD**, received her baccalaureate from St. Joseph College, her master's degree from The Catholic University of America, and her doctoral degree from Teacher's College, Columbia University. She taught at Lehman College in New York City and at the University of Wisconsin in Oshkosh. She is currently Associate Professor at the Philip Y. Hahn School of Nursing, University of San Diego, San Diego, California. Dr. Rauckhorst is nationally recognized for her leadership as past President of the National Organization of Nurse Practitioners.

**Shirlee Ann Stokes, RN, EdD, FAAN,** received her baccalaureateand master's degrees from Ohio State University, and her doctoral degree from Teacher's College, Columbia University. She taught at Lehman College in New York City and at Case Western Reserve University in Cleveland, Ohio. She is currently Associate Dean at the Lienhard School of Nursing at Pace University in Pleasantville, New York. Dr. Stokes is nationally recognized for her development of the Stokes/Gordon Scale to measure life stress in older adults.

Second Edition

# HEALTH ASSESSMENT of the OLDER INDIVIDUAL

**Mathy Doval Mezey,** RN, EdD, FAAN

**Louise Hartnett Rauckhorst,** RNC, ANP, EdD

**Shirlee Ann Stokes,** RN, EdD, FAAN

 Springer Publishing Company • New York

Springer Publishing Company, Inc.
536 Broadway
New York, NY 10012

First edition published in 1980

93 94 95 96 97 / 5 4 3 2

---

**Library of Congress Cataloging-in-Publication Data**

Mezey, Mathy Doval.
    Health assessment of the older individual / Mathy D. Mezey, Louise
H. Rauckhorst, Shirlee A. Stokes. — 2nd ed.
       p.    cm. — (Springer series on geriatric nursing)
    Includes bibliographical references and index.
    ISBN 0-8261-2902-1
    1. Geriatric nursing.  2. Nursing assessment.  I. Rauckhorst,
Louise Hartnett.  II. Stokes, Shirlee Ann.  III. Title.  IV. Series.
    [DNLM: 1. Geriatric Nursing.  WY 152 M617h]
    RC954.M49   1993
    618.97'075—dc20
    DNLM/DLC
    for Library of Congress                          92-49574
                                              CIP

---

Printed in the United States of America

*It is as though walking down Shaftesbury Avenue as a fairly young man I was suddenly kidnapped, rushed into a theater and made to don the gray hair, the wrinkles and the other attributes of age, then wheeled on stage. Behind the appearance of age I am the same person, with the same thoughts, as when I was younger.*

—J. B. Priestley (at age 79, on being asked—on the occasion of publication of his 99th work—what it's like being old)
*Time Magazine*, September 24, 1973

# Contents

# Preface

The second edition of this book has been revised to provide practitioners with a concise, up-to-date reference text on health assessment of elderly clients. It is intended for use by practitioners who work in diverse health settings in a variety of health fields.

The book presents normal age changes, common deviations from the normal, and common health problems. All chapters of the prior edition have been updated to reflect the changing parameters of health assessment. The chapter on musculoskeletal assessment has been expanded to include a section on falls assessment. The chapter on community and home assessment has been expanded to include information for practitioners on assessment of a nursing home. The new chapters on functional, nutritional, and mental health assessment and on laboratory values reflect the expanding body of knowledge in these fields. Because many of these health assessment areas overlap, the reader will need to view the chapters in the context of the whole book in order to gain a comprehensive view of health assessment of older persons.

The information presented in this text will enable the practitioner to assist older persons in achieving and maintaining optimal health, to identify older individuals and groups who have a high-risk profile for health problems, and to identify specific deviations from the normal and the resulting impact on lifestyle and activities of daily living.

This book presupposes basic knowledge of health history taking and the physical examination process. The emphasis here is on specific adaptations in focus and technique in history taking and physical examination when obtaining database information from older people. The reader may need to refer to basic texts in anatomy, physiology, pathophysiology, as well as physical examination and history-taking techniques for further background.

Each of the three authors contributed equally to the book; the order of their names was determined in a random drawing.

MDM
LHR
SAS

ix

# The Role of Assessment in the Care of the Older Person

The focus of this book is on comprehensive health assessment of the older person. Older people manifest specific normal age changes and health problems that differ from those experienced by younger people. These differences are the focal point of this text.

A health care encounter has four components: assessment, planning, implementation, and evaluation. This book focuses mainly on the assessment phase of the encounter with the elderly client. The ultimate purpose of the text is to assist nurses to plan, deliver, and evaluate quality care to the elderly. The knowledge base needed to formulate a comprehensive health plan for the older person is extensive and the need to incorporate new knowledge into clinical practice is continuous.

Collecting health-related information about an individual is necessarily purposeful and a holistic perspective is essential for formulation of a comprehensive health plan. To accomplish this goal the practitioner needs to understand the biologic as well as sociocultural, psychologic, and spiritual nature of older people. For example, if one knows that an elderly person with Parkinsonian tremors is a practicing Jew, the practitioner can then inquire as to the implications of hand tremors in regard to lighting the Friday evening Sabbath candles.

The American Nurses' Association *Standards of Geriatric Nursing Practice* (1986) and guidelines for assessment developed by the American

College of Physicians (1988) emphasize the importance of the assessment process. Standard 3 of the ANA Standards, for example, states: "The nurse observes and interprets minimal as well as gross signs and symptoms associated with both normal aging and pathologic changes and institutes appropriate nursing measures" (p. 6). There is evidence that geriatric nurses and physicians hold highly congruent opinions as to what constitutes appropriate assessment of the elderly (Mezey, Lavizzo-Mourey, Brunswick, & Taylor, 1992; Lavizzo-Mourey, Mezey, & Taylor, 1991).

The assessment process itself encompasses three phases: the collection of information or data; the analysis of the data; and the formulation of judgments. The first phase, collection of information about an individual, can be accomplished in a variety of ways. To avoid gaps, data collection is best accomplished by a practitioner who has an organized plan. In this book data collection methods are presented in a specific systematic way. First, the interview is used to collect the client profile, past health history, and review of systems data. Second, the physical examination skills of inspection, palpation, percussion, and auscultation are used to gather further information. Third, data about the community and home setting are collected. Finally, recommendations as to the collection of laboratory data are presented.

In the second, or analysis, phase of assessment the information gathered is processed and sorted in the health provider's mind. Data analysis is an intellectual process. It is at this point that the practitioner organizes the available knowledge within a theoretical framework to determine the significance and ramifications of the information gathered, or to determine the need for additional information. For example, a practitioner whose framework is to focus on the strengths rather than the deficits associated with aging, may want to accompany an older person on a walk to see how well they maneuver steps and other obstacles. The greater the practitioner's knowledge base, the more effectively and completely information is processed. The content regarding normal and abnormal processes of aging and age changes provided in this book should aid the nurse in this analysis of data.

The final phase and outcome of the assessment process is the formulation of a professional judgment. Judgments include identification of strengths and/or health limitations of the individual, and what treatment strategies appear most beneficial and most feasible. These judgements are then shared with the older person and the family and, through a process of clarification and discussion, mutual goals are formulated, priorities are set, and a plan of care is developed.

At the present time there is a tentative nature to existing theories of aging and the fund of knowledge regarding the elderly client. The number of older people in our society has increased markedly over the last century. The population over 65 years of age in 1900 was 3 million, in contrast to more than 33 million in 1990. As of 1990, older people made up 1 in 8 of the total population. By the year 2030 older people will make up 20% or 1 in 5 of the total population (U.S. Bureau of the Census, 1990).

Concern about the elderly, unheard of in 1900 when life expectancy was 45 years, is now a daily source of discussion in the lay and professional press. Scientists are only now beginning to understand the process of aging (Rowe, 1985). As our understanding increases, methods for altering the course of aging may emerge. Societal changes have already resulted in revision of modes of living for the elderly, and communities are developing special services to meet the needs of the older individual.

In using this text, the reader should keep in mind that it is difficult to apply a concept of normalcy to the older individual. In providing care it is often difficult to distinguish between what is "normal" and what is prevalent. For example, 25 years ago diminished vision from cataracts was regarded as a normal concomitant of aging. Today, cataracts are identified as abnormal findings amenable to treatment.

Mortality and morbidity in older people are currently attributable primarily to accidents and chronic disease. The leading causes of death are vascular disease, diabetes, hypertension, and cancer. Future research and medical advances will have a direct and indirect effect on mortality and morbidity rates. One recent medical advance, control of hypertension, has already decreased morbidity and mortality among American blacks, and thus helped to narrow the difference in mortality rates between nonwhites and whites. Other advances in health care that have the potential to substantially affect mortality rates among future cohorts of older people include primary and secondary prevention of dementia, prevention and improved treatment of cancer, prevention of osteoporosis, and control of the effects of environmental pollutants such as cigarette smoke and radiation. Research into chronic debilitating disease, although not necessarily leading to curative therapies, may improve the quality of life, and indirectly affect mortality. For example, medication to alleviate the pain of arthritis would substantially improve functional status and decrease social isolation and prevalence of injury.

Rising levels of income and education will also affect the health of future cohorts of older people and will alter our concept of normal aging. Socioeconomic status and poor education are negatively correlated with mortality in the elderly. Mortality rates are highest for nonfarm laborers and lowest for professionals. An intellectual lifestyle is associated with increased longevity. Based on these facts, mortality rates for today's cohort of younger people should be lower when they reach old age than for the population that is presently over 65.

Because their first professional encounter with older people is often in hospitals and nursing homes, neophyte nurses can easily believe the stereotypes of most older people as helpless, sick, and intellectually impaired. These stereotypes are not confirmed by facts. Most older people are not sick. While they are hospitalized more frequently and for longer periods than their younger counterparts, for the most part older people are active and functioning in society. Three-fourths of the population of older people are totally independent and lead their lives without needing help of any kind (National Medical Expenditure Survey, 1990). Only 5% of the population over 65 are so severely disabled that they are bedfast or homebound (Strumpf & Stevenson, 1991).

Comprehensive assessment encompasses not only the older person but also involves information about family and community supports. From the moment older people talk about a symptom with a family member or friend, to the time when they need help in recovering from an acute or chronic episode of illness, a complete understanding of the elderly person's health care needs cannot be achieved in the absence of consideration of their family and lay supports (Brody, 1990). Aspects of family assessment are considered within each chapter of this book, and especially in the chapter on home and community assessment.

With the expanding range of health care practice, health assessment is now carried out in many nontraditional settings: group practices and systems of managed care, satellite health care facilities in apartment buildings and senior centers, and in continuing care retirement communities. The geriatric practitioner tries to encounter clients in their own settings and, wherever possible, assesses older individuals in the environment in which they live. It is not unusual for the geriatric nurse to organize health fairs to screen large numbers of older people, or to receive referrals from the clergy who see older people in their homes. It is the intent of this book to assist the practitioner to consider a broad and comprehensive framework for this practice, so that issues of greatest concern to the elderly and their families are adequately addressed.

# REFERENCES

American College of Physicians Health and Public Policy Committee (1988). Comprehensive Functional Assessment for Elderly Patients. *Annals of Internal Medicine, 33*, 70–72.
American Nurses' Association (1986). *Standards of geriatric nursing practice.* Kansas City, MO: Author.

Brody, E. (1990). *Women in the middle: Their parent-care years.* New York: Springer Publishing Co.

Lavizzo-Mourey, R., Mezey, M., & Taylor, L. (1991). The admission assessment in teaching nursing homes. *Journal of the American Geriatric Society, 39,* 268–74.

Mezey, A., Lavizzo-Mourey, R., Brunswick, J., & Taylor, L. (1992). The assessment of nursing home patients. *The Nurse Practitioner, 17,* 50–61.

National Medical Expenditure Survey. (1990). *Functional status of the noninstitutionalized elderly: Estimates of ADL and IADL difficulties.* (Department of Health & Human Services; DHHS Publication No. 90-3462.) Washington, DC: U.S. Government Printing Office.

Rowe, J. (1985). Health care of the elderly. *New England Journal of Medicine, 312,* 827–35.

Strumpf, N., & Stevenson, C. (1991). Breaking new ground in elder care: Practice, research and education. In Aiken, L. H., & Fagin, C. M. *Charting nursing's future: Agenda for the 1990s.* Philadelphia: J. B. Lippincott.

U.S. Bureau of the Census. (1990). *Projections of the population of the United States by age, sex, and race: 1983 to 2080.* (Publication P-25, No. 952). Washington, DC: U.S. Government Printing Office.

# 2

# Growth and Development of the Older Person

Although this text emphasizes the biologic and psychologic changes that occur with age, no assessment of the older person is complete without a consideration of the individual as a functioning whole. Unfortunately there is a tendency to describe older people in such a way as to maximize the similarities between them and minimize their differences. Older people are often described as being homogeneous in appearance and having undifferentiated lifestyles. This is an inaccurate picture of aging. People tend to remain heterogeneous and highly individualistic into old age, and they continue to have what deBeauvoir describes as a "plurality of experience" (deBeauvior, 1972, p. 281).

When gathering the data base, therefore, the practitioner must be cognizant of the older person's unique history and health needs. Knowledge of the growth and development changes that occur as part of the aging process is a helpful framework for the practitioner working with the elderly. This chapter is an attempt to explore current issues and knowledge of growth and development that have relevance to the health assessment of older people.

## THEORIES OF AGING

Aging can be described as a result of the human organism's continuing interaction with biologic, psychologic, and sociocultural change from one point in time to another. A multiplicity of theories exists as to why and how aging occurs (Cristotalo, 1990).

Current theories of why aging occurs are varied and highly speculative. The "wear and tear" theory suggests that with increasing age the body's physiologic functions deteriorate to the point that they are unable to sustain life. These deteriorations are thought to occur as a result of people's interaction with the external environment and because of cellular loss and degeneration resulting from the lifelong attempts of the body to maintain internal homeostasis. Proponents of this theory suggest that, as physiologic decrements increase over time, the individual becomes less able to tolerate stress and becomes increasingly vulnerable to disease.

A second theory suggests that life span is genetically controlled and that human beings have a maximal life expectancy of approximately 120 years. Aging might result primarily from changes in the body's immune system and/or endocrine system, or the increase in exposure to and production of free radicals. Decline in either the immune and/or endocrine systems slows the regenerative and adaptive abilities of the human.

Recent investigations of "slow viruses" have led some scientists to suggest a viral theory of aging. Slow viruses may enter the body at any time in the life cycle and begin to affect cells, such as those in the brain and nervous system, after an incubation period of several decades. Because slow viruses can affect the immune system, it has been suggested that this theory may be closely related to the immunological theory of aging.

It is not yet possible to distinguish which age changes occur as a true result of the aging process and which manifestations of aging occur as the result of a variety of environmental and physical factors. Current knowledge about older people's development is derived from comparisons of past and current groups of older and younger people. The life experience of people currently in their twenties, however, is completely different from that of the group of people who are 65 and over. The education, nutrition, health care, exposure to pollutants, and life stresses of the two groups vary enormously. This concept of differences between cohort groups, that is, groups of people who are born at different points in time, has wide implications for the health practitioner.

## BIOLOGIC CHANGES

In general, the physical changes that occur with aging constitute a continuation of declines that began in middle age. Older people have diminished adaptive qualities. They are less able to maintain and regain homeostasis. This decreased adaptive quality is especially marked if the individual undergoes biologic and psychologic stress. For example, when an older person develops an infection, the body temperature does not rise as rapidly or markedly as might be expected in a younger individual; and once having risen, the older person's temperature takes longer to return to normal. The increased susceptibility of older people to hypothermia is another example of altered homeostasis experienced with aging.

Alterations in physical appearance that occur with aging are generally due to connective tissue changes. The parenchymal tissue of the body decreases more rapidly in comparison with the supportive substances, such as collagen fibers. The thinning and fragmentation of elastin fibers accounts for many of the changes evident in the skin of older people.

There is a decrease in function of multiple organ systems, including a decrease in cardiac output, vital capacity, muscle strength, and renal blood flow. These changes account for the diminished basal metabolic rate of older people and a concomitant, frequently occurring weight gain and change in the fat/lean ratio. Factors such as poor nutritional status and diminished vision, hearing, and taste further contribute to the generalized slowing of pace and decreased capacity for physical work experienced by many older people.

## PSYCHOLOGIC CHANGES

Psychologic changes that occur with aging have cognitive, affective, and psychomotor components. Biologic, psychologic, and social aging do not necessarily occur simultaneously. Psychologic changes can precede or follow biologic and social age changes.

The major developmental tasks of old age can be categorized as follows:

- Maintaining independence
- Relinquishing power
- Coping with losses
- Initiating a life review process
- Developing a philosophical perspective on life

Several theorists have identified additional life tasks and crises of aging. Erikson et al. describes the 65-year-old individual as one who is completing the Psychosocial Stage of Care. In this stage, the middle-aged and young older adult struggles with generativity versus stagnation. Somewhere in the early seventies, the older individual enters the stage of wisdom (Erikson, 1963).

This final stage is a time when all earlier experiences are integrated and the outcome is characterized as either integrity or despair (Erikson, Erikson, & Kivnick, 1986). Peck has identified the tasks of old age as: ego differentiation versus work role preoccupation; body transcendence versus body preoccupation; and ego transcendence versus ego preoccupation (Peck, 1968). The common factor identified in the life tasks attributed to old age is the need for the individual to adjust to declines in all levels of functioning while also maintaining the self and continuing to grow as a person.

## PERSONALITY

In general, while the personality as a whole tends to become increasingly rigid with age, most personality variables remain relatively stable throughout life. It is especially important for the practitioner to determine the history of the client's personality characteristics over the life cycle prior to assuming that current personality manifestations constitute an age change.

In many instances increased anxiety concerning health exerts a strong influence on the older person's behavior. Aging requires the individual to face the issue of declining physical health. Many older people manifest the phenomenon of body monitoring, that is, the increased attention paid to physical changes and bodily functions. Whether this body preoccupation becomes the overwhelming motivation of later life is a major developmental task for the older person to resolve.

The older person must also resolve the task of accommodating to the death of family members and peers and to his or her own impending death. Many elderly people go through a process of reminiscing and life review. Through this normal and highly therapeutic process older clients relate past accomplishments and occurrences in an effort to verbalize to themselves and to others the meaning of their life.

## COGNITIVE FUNCTIONING

While cognitive function tends to decrease with age, under normal circumstances the changes have little effect on day-to-day functioning. The change is most apparent in individuals who have sharply constricted their integration with the physical and psychosocial environment. The issue of change in intelligence over the life cycle is complicated and as yet unresolved. Recent studies suggest that intelligence may not show a decline if it is measured with a test that contains items specific to older people. Ideally, when cognitive aging is successful, the older individual passes from abstract thinking to post formal thought. Post formal thought is a higher level of reasoning whereby the individual places the event into the context of total life experiences. The wisdom ascribed to the older individual is an example of post formal thought (Sinnott, 1989).

While vocabulary increases over the life cycle, the older person has an altered capacity to acquire and retain new information and learn new tasks. These deficits can be minimized in an environment that provides opportunity for repetition, manipulation, and multiple trials, and where time restriction is not a factor.

## AFFECTIVE CHANGES

Psychologic changes also influence the individual's self-perception. In addition to observable biologic and psychologic changes, aging is a state of mind perceived internally by the individual. Most misconceptions and misunderstandings regarding aging probably stem from discrepancies between how the older person and others view the aging process.

Most older people report a general satisfaction with their current life stage. Self-ratings indicate that most elderly perceive strong points about themselves, see themselves as having moral worth, and are no more preoccupied with death than are younger adults. Many older people are concerned about the quality of the years of life remaining until death. They often speak of the number of "good years" that remain rather than the actual number of years of life anticipated.

How older people view their health is one of the best predictors of life satisfaction. When older people talk about health, they are primarily referring to their functional ability. If people feel that they can fulfill functions related to maintaining independence and social roles, they will usually say that their health is good, irrespective of the degree of physiologic impairment. Despite the increased incidence of illness and hospitalizations experienced by older people, most rate their health as good. In general, older people see themselves as healthier than do health professionals. They tend to rate their health as good, irrespective of the number of times they see a doctor, the amount of medication taken, or current objective professional designation of health status.

Another major aspect of the older person's self-perception is age identification. Age identification implies a relationship between the individual and a model with which the individual feels a likeness. In general, only 30% to 40% of people over 65 will call themselves old (Tuckman & Lorge, 1953).

> Chronological age seems to be a poor index of aging and may serve as only a convenient means of ordering developmental data. It appears that age-identification, rather than actual age, constrains older people to recognize changes in themselves, and to perceive that the attitudes of others toward them have changed (Peters, 1971, p. 72).

Subjective age identification is particularly significant for older people, since it gives a clue as to how they feel they should behave. A person who thinks of him or herself as old will tend to assume the characteristics of being "old."

## SOCIOCULTURAL CHANGES

Social age reflects performance of age-specific roles. Social age can be a state of development or a status confirmed by a social group. Aging seems to bring with it a decrease in social alternatives and options. In general there is an involuntary constriction of social roles—retirement or death of friends and family members as well as diminution in affiliative roles. Income reduction and illness may lead to a shrinking use of life space, which further contributes to social isolation.

While older people tend to be more dependent on others and are high receivers of family assistance, it is not true that most of the aged are unable to care for themselves. The great majority of older people live in their own homes, many as heads of households. There is no evidence that disengagement occurs as an inevitable counterpart to growing old. Rather, the pattern of social participation seems to remain consistent throughout the life cycle. Older people who have led active lives during adulthood report having "no free time" following retirement, and they describe a wide variety of social and volunteer activities. On the other hand, the person who has been isolated during middle age will tend to continue this noninteractive pattern into old age. The importance of family roles also shows a wide range of variability. Although some people report that family ties serve as the basis of most social interactions, others do not see family relationships as central to their social activities.

Older people are often described by others as wanting to remain by themselves, but most of the elderly voice a strong desire to interact with younger people. Indeed, Activity Theory supports the notion that life satisfaction is greater in individuals who remain involved in personal and social pursuits (Havighurst, & Albrecht, 1953). While many of the aged seem to prefer age-segregated housing, most express a desire to communicate with younger adults.

The practitioner should remember that society can and does ascribe to the aged those roles and privileges commensurate with its underlying philosophy, irrespective of the facts. Although the biologic changes that occur with age are relatively constant for all societies, the status of older people varies markedly from one society to another.

In our society, people often devalue and define older people as noncontributing and nonproductive. Examples of this are abundant in the media today. Words used in literature to describe older people often highlight their frailties and negative characteristics. Visions of the frightful old witch in children's fairy tales or jokes about a dirty old man imply a reliance on the benevolence of society. Many older people resent this labeling and are actively working to accurately portray themselves (Covey, 1988).

## NURSING IMPLICATIONS

Age, like sex and race, is a biologically defined human difference that affects all aspects of an interactive process. It is important to assess how well individuals have adapted to their perceived age changes. Similarly, it is important to determine the extent to which people are accomplishing the developmental tasks of aging.

As people age, they perceive that others react positively or negatively to them. Practitioners working with older people bring to the interaction all their stereotypes and perceptions of how someone who is old should act, feel, and think. This process, of course, occurs in all interpersonal relationships. It has special significance, however, when considering the health assessment of the older person because of the predominantly negative stereotypes that most people have about the elderly. If, for example, the practitioner has the stereotype that older people are depressed, unhappy, and dependent, this will obviously affect the interactive process and interfere with the collection and interpretation of an accurate data base. Therefore, practitioners need to become especially aware of their feelings and attitudes toward older people prior to undertaking the assessment process.

In summary, the practitioner's awareness of growth and development enhances the health assessment. While knowledge of the developmental changes that occur with age is helpful when thinking about older people, the practitioner must respect the uniqueness of the life experience of each individual older adult.

## REFERENCES

deBeauvoir, S. (1972). *The coming of age*. New York: G.P. Putnam's Sons.

Cristofalo, V. J. (1990). Biological mechanisms of aging: An overview. In Hazzard, W. R., Andres, R., Bierman, E. L., & Blass, J. P. (Eds.). *Principles of geriatric medicine and gerontology*. New York: McGraw-Hill.

Covey, H. C. (1988, June). Historical terminology used to represent older people. *The Gerontologist, 28*(3), 291, 297.

Erikson, E. H., Erikson, J. M., & Kivnick, H. Q. (1986). *Vital involvement in old age*, (pp. 54–104). New York: W. W. Norton & Co.

Erikson, E. H. (1963). Generativity and ego Integrity. In Neugarten, B. L. (Ed.). *Middle age and aging*. Chicago: University of Chicago Press.

Havighurst, F. J., & Albrecht, R. (1953). *Older people*. New York: Longmans Green.

Peck, R. C. (1968). Psychological development in the second half of life. In Neugarten, B. L. (Ed.). *Middle age and aging* (pp. 90–99). Chicago: University of Chicago Press.

Peters, G. R. (1971, Winter). Self-conceptions of the aged: Age Identification and aging. *The Gerontologist, 11*(4), 69–73.

Sinnott, J. D. (1989). Life-span relativistic post formal thought: Methodology and data from everyday problem-solving studies. In Commons, M. L., Sinnott, J. D., Richards, F. A., & Arman, C. (Eds.). *Adult development comparisons and applications of developmental models. Vol. 1*, (pp. 239–278). New York: New York Praeger.

Tuckman, J., & Lorge, I. (1953). Classification of the self as young, middle aged, or old. *Geriatrics, 9*, 534.

## SUGGESTED READINGS

Bengtson, V., & Schaie, K. W. (1989). *The course of later life: Research and reflections*. New York: Springer Publishing Co.

Busse, E. W., & Maddox, G. L. (1985). *The Duke Longitudinal Studies of Normal Aging, 1955–1980*. New York: Springer Publishing Co.

Binstock, R. H., & George, L. K. (Eds). (1990). *Handbook of aging and the social sciences*. New York: Van Nostrand & Reinhold.

Eliopoulos, C. (1990). *Caring for the elderly in diverse care settings*. Philadelphia: J. B. Lippincott.

Hazzard, W. R., Andres, P., Bierman, E. L., & Blass, J. P. (Eds.). (1990). *Principles of geriatric medicine and gerontology*. New York: McGraw-Hill, Inc.

Kalish, R. A. (1981). *Late adulthood: Perspectives on human development*. Monterey, CA: Brooks-Cole Publishing Co.

Kuhlen, R. (1968). Developmental changes in motivation during the adult years. In Neugarten, B. L. (Ed.), *Middle age and aging.* Chicago: University of Chicago Press.

Lee, R. J. (1976, March). Self images of the elderly. *Nursing Clinics of North America, 11*(1), 119–124.

Palmore, E. (1988). Facts on Aging. New York, Springer Publishing Co.

Schaie, K. W., Campbell, R., Meredith, W., & Rawlings, S. (Eds.). (1988). *Methodological issues in aging research.* New York: Springer Publishing Co.

# 3

# Interviewing for the Health History

The purpose of this chapter is to discuss methods for adapting usual interviewing techniques when eliciting a history from older people. As with clients of any age, the collection of a relevant data base begins by obtaining a complete and detailed health history. The history should serve as your "window" to the client. In addition to the past and present health status, this history should include the client's perception of him- or herself, detailing perceived strengths and weaknesses. The history becomes the basis for interpreting physical findings as well as community, home, and laboratory data, and suggests appropriate plans of care.

The prevalence of certain diseases and disorders in the older population should be taken into consideration in evaluating older people's symptoms. The entire health assessment process, beginning with the health history, should identify opportunities for health promotion. It should also screen for diseases or impairments with a higher incidence in the elderly and for which preventive measures and/or early detection and treatment have been shown to have a significant effect on morbidity and mortality. These would include heart disease, stroke, colo-rectal and skin cancer, fractures, dental and foot problems, and auditory and visual impairments (U.S. Department of Health and Human Services, 1991).

As the various pieces of health assessment information are gathered, the health care provider's knowledge of the diseases and functional problems that more commonly occur in the elderly will suggest the range of possible/probable medical, functional, and psychosocial problems that need to be addressed and prioritized in developing the plan of care (Gallo, Reichel, & Anderson, 1988). If the older client, family member, or the past medical record reveals numerous complaints and problems, the care provider may feel overwhelmed. The essential task is to identify and remain clear about which problems need to be addressed at once and which ones can wait. It is often most helpful to focus on the special medical, functional, and/or psychosocial problems that prompted the visit. However, keeping track of all the older individual's coexisting, and often interacting, problems is also important. Management of priority problems cannot be safely planned and implemented in a vacuum—the possible positive and negative interactions of multiple medical, functional, and psychosocial problems must always be considered (Gallo et al., 1988).

# FACTORS AFFECTING COMMUNICATION

## The Interviewer

The young adult may have stereotypes about the elderly that affect communication. Because of the age discrepancy the younger practitioner may feel that the older client will be uncomfortable answering questions of a personal nature, anticipating a response like, "You have no business asking such questions. You're young enough to be my grandchild." In fact, these stereotypes are not supported by current research. The greatest desire of older people is for relationships with others. They are anxious to interact with younger people, but they also fear rejection.

Younger adults see older clients as different from themselves. For example, calling the elderly by their first name or by a pet name reflects a stereotype of the older adult as childlike, dependent, or senile. Address the older person in terms indicating equality and respect. Another common assumption of younger adults is that the aged are dependent and preoccupied with death. In truth, most older people live in their own homes or apartments and are concerned with customary activities of everyday life, such as paying expenses, negotiating transportation, and shopping.

The ability of the interviewer to elicit data will depend on the interviewer's comfort in asking the questions. As competency and expertise increase, the practitioner will become more comfortable in asking personal questions and in forming relationships with older adults.

## The Client

Several factors may influence the completeness of the history obtained from an older person. Older people differ in their willingness to divulge their life histories. If you are a stranger, they may be suspicious, especially since paranoia is more frequent in the older age group. It may take repeated contacts and careful explanations to allay fears. Under appropriate conditions, however, most older people are anxious to share their histories with a concerned and interested person.

Older people may not understand the purpose of a complete history. Many elderly have had little contact with the health care delivery system. They may fail to see the relevance to their current health of questions regarding habits, previous life experiences, or social status. The practitioner needs to explain the relevance of certain personal information in planning the overall health promotion and maintenance for the individual.

For many people over 65 the verbal tradition is not customary. A large number are foreign-born and have not completed high school. Approximately one-third of the urban elderly live in relative isolation, having only brief daily contacts with people, and have therefore become less verbal. For these individuals, the practitioner needs to use focused interviewing techniques in eliciting information. In addition, older people may be unfamiliar with common health-related terminology or they may attach their own unique meanings to terms such as stroke, heart attack, or constipation. It is helpful to obtain consensual validation of shared meanings throughout the interview.

Older people are aware of declines that occur with aging and may be hesitant to have some of their fears confirmed. They are concerned that illness may result in loss of independence or lead to institutionalization. They may be aware of memory loss or recent events associated with decreased ability to concentrate and they may be embarrassed to discuss some topics because of this. On the other hand, some older people may erroneously attribute their symptoms to normal aging and, therefore, tend to underreport them. Being as supportive and reassuring as possible throughout the interview will be especially helpful.

When healthy older persons are not stressed, physiologic changes due to normal aging often are not significant enough to be clinically detected. The number of current diseases and medications is a better predictor of symptom prevalence than is age (Hale, Perkins, & May et al. 1986). Exercise caution about attributing signs and symptoms to aging (which is irreversible) rather than to health problems that might be amenable to treatment (Brody, Kliban, & Moles, 1983). In addition, the elderly may present with different signs and symptoms of certain diseases than younger people. For example, they are more likely than younger people to be afebrile with pneumococcal bacteremia (Norman, Grahn, & Yoshikawa, 1985), to be pain-free with myocardial infarction, pneumonia, pulmonary embolism, perforated peptic ulcer, or acute cholecystitis, or to be lethargic rather than hyperactive with hyperthyroidism (Caird, 1981). They are also more likely to have nonspecific complaints such as falling, weakness, or syncope with a variety of specific diseases.

It often takes time and patience to identify the priorities of the older client's concerns and to establish the actual reason for the visit. They frequently present with multiple complaints (an average of three to five symptoms) rather than with one chief complaint (Brody et al., 1983). Symptoms elicited during the health history may be due to the synergistic effect of two or more chronic diseases, or an acute process superimposed on a chronic one. Also, the symptoms of one disease may mask the expected symptoms of another. For example, an elderly person with restricted mobility due to arthritis may not report increasing dyspnea with worsening congestive heart failure.

It is important to assess the impact of irreversible chronic disorders on the older client's ability to function since some effects that can significantly impair the individual's ability to function (for example, incontinence) may be reversible. The complaints of older adults or their family members may also be unstated, vague, or not in the usual mold— for example, "Dad is just not himself" or "Mom doesn't cook anymore." In these cases, the interviewer will need to remain alert to clues throughout the assessment process that can help to pinpoint the nature and etiology of the problem(s).

## The Flow of the Interview

To initiate positive communication at the start of the interview it is important to establish eye contact, to address the older client by his or her last name, and to use touch appropriately (for example, shake hands or touch the client's shoulder in a caring way), while briefly explaining what is to be accomplished during the visit. Respect the older client's personal space and identify the presence of significant auditory and/or visual deficits early in the interview so that these barriers to communication can be overcome. The client should be wearing his or her glasses and/or hearing aid, if appropriate. Ask early in the interview whether the client is able to hear. If the client has a hearing impairment, directly face the client at a close but comfortable distance and speak slowly with clear articulation and a well-modulated voice, resisting the tendency to raise its pitch and volume, since this usually decreases the older client's speech comprehension. Stay alert for signs of communication problems such as reluctance to continue, lack of eye contact, or signs of physical discomfort or fatigue.

Several factors may affect the practitioner's ability to control the flow of the interview. The elderly often have long and complicated personal and medical histories. The 80-year-old has more to tell than the 30-year-old. Some older individuals are reluctant to provide information, whereas others are eager to share at length. Older clients may give too much data in an effort to be complete, or because they enjoy recounting happenings of long ago that are not directly pertinent to the goals of the present interview. When they seem to ramble on, older clients will usually not take offense at being gently interrupted and guided back to the health history.

The respectful sharing of some reminiscences can, however, both increase understanding of the client's past and values, and increase rapport. A universal concern of the elderly is life review and integration of past events with current situations. One question may lead to a chain of thoughts, and it may be difficult to keep the client on the topic. The life review can serve as an excellent source of data relevant to multiple areas of the health history.

It is helpful to set a time limit at the beginning of the interview. A statement such as, "I am going to spend the next 45 minutes asking you about yourself, your past life, and your current health," is usually sufficient. This statement also helps to orient the client to the interview and deal with the potential problem of decreased time perception.

The older person may be slow in responding to questions. Reaction time to verbal stimuli is typically lengthened; the interviewer needs to allow sufficient time for the client to formulate responses. Attempts to hurry the response lead to anxiety, confusion, and embarrassment, with a consequent sketchy data base. The time scheduled for interviewing an older person is necessarily long. If a full history is indicated, it may be advisable to gather data over several sessions.

The way questions are stated is also very important. Older clients are more likely to use the vocabulary of their time and not add new words. Contemporary colloquialisms or slang are often not understood. Questions should be short and concise, and the number of words should be restricted to essential components. One piece of information should be asked in each question. The interviewer should ask questions that will serve a multiple purpose to elicit information in the quickest possible way. Focused interview techniques may facilitate responses, especially if the client demonstrates difficulty with abstract thinking. Use of techniques such as clarifying and summation help to assure validity of information. When the client's response seems unclear, rephrasing the question is helpful. Practice will help to facilitate the obtaining of information in a short period of time.

If the older client has a significant memory deficit, family members and/or other alternate data sources can be used, with the client's permission. Even in these cases, however, the interviewer should always obtain as much information directly from the older client as possible—in particular, what they perceive to be their main health-related problem(s). If family members are present at the interview, they should be directed to refrain from answering questions unless they are asked to do so (Starer & Libow, 1990, p. 154). The interviewer may also have an opportunity to speak with the family while the older client undresses for the physical examination, or at another time. Additional time needs to be scheduled not only for the history, but also for the physical examination, since responding to physical examination directions as well as undressing and moving to and from the examining table, take longer.

## The Setting

The environment should be as free as possible of extraneous noise and interruptions. The older person will need some time to become acquainted with the surroundings at the beginning of the interview. Arthritis and other disabilities may make sitting for long periods painful; the chair for the client should be comfortable, of adequate height, and have sturdy arms. Time intervals should be allotted for movement.

Sensory deficits further impede interviewing and require modification of the environment. A well-lit room will help to compensate for visual deficiencies. Diminished hearing is common, especially in higher frequencies. The room should be as quiet as possible, because outside noises tend to make it more difficult for the client to respond.

The morning is the most appropriate time to schedule the health history. Fatigue will contribute to decrease in mental functioning. In addition, older people are concerned about their safety, and often do not like late afternoon appointments, particularly in the winter.

## OBTAINING THE CLIENT PROFILE

One of the first judgments the practitioner must make is to determine the reliability of information obtained from the older client. Unfamiliar surroundings can contribute to confusion. The elderly also have a high incidence of depression, which may be confused with dementia. When the client seems unable to give a clear and complete history, the interviewer needs to be familiar with the signs and symptoms of confusion, dementia, and depression. If confusion is suspected, questions should be asked to determine orientation to time, place, person, and present and past events (see Chapter 11). Evidence of dementia should not automatically stop history-taking with the older client. Demented individuals are often able to report useful information, even though they are unable to place historical events in their correct time sequence. If necessary, family can be consulted to further determine reliability of the client and to supplement the history. A home visit can also provide important data as to how well the client is able to respond to questions in familiar surroundings (see Chapter 13).

Data obtained from the client profile provides information not only on the level of functioning but also on life satisfaction. Because of our present lack of knowledge of what constitutes "normal functioning" in the elderly, the client's perceptions and self-evaluation are of special significance. In all areas it is important to determine what the older person is able to do and how the person feels about what he or she is able to do.

In general, most older people are realistic about their health. Shanas and colleagues report: "The self-evaluation that old people make of their health is highly correlated with their reports of restriction in mobility, their sensory impairments, and their overall incapacity scores. In general, if any old person says his health is poor, he has a physical basis for this self-judgment (Shanas, Townsend, Wedderburn et al., 1968, p. 215).

It is important to recognize, however, that the meaning of "being healthy" varies greatly in older people. If anything, older people tend to be "health optimists," overestimating their health and minimizing symptoms. This is especially true of the older person who is able to carry out activities of daily living to his or her satisfaction. Others may not report symptoms because they assume these are age appropriate and therefore of no interest to the practitioner. For example, older clients may not mention the pain of arthritis, since they would not see this as a health problem in the same manner as a younger adult.

In contrast, some elderly adults are "health pessimists." These are people who have not completed one developmental task of aging, which according to Peck (1968), concerns itself with body transcendence. Instead, these people are preoccupied with their bodies and exaggerate and dwell on the physical declines that occur with aging. The practitioner should try to assess whether the client is a "health optimist" or a "health pessimist," since this will greatly influence the way in which the self and health problems are perceived.

Psychosocial factors may influence the health status of older people, even more than they do that of younger clients (Burrage, Dixon, & Sehy, 1991). It is important to determine who the individual lives with and what supports (family or others) are available to provide assistance if needed. It is also important to determine the number and types of social contacts. Is the client satisfied with his or her social contacts? Does he or she get out of the house daily? Weekly? Monthly? Does a pet play an important role in the elder's life? Does he or she have a friend or relative to rely upon in case of an emergency? Frequently older people are afraid of dying alone and of not being discovered for several days. Psychosocial data are often extremely helpful in planning effective interventions; for example, in regard to weight loss due to undernutrition, alleviating social isolation and taking care of poor finances and/ or lack of transportation may be more important than the provision of nutritional counseling.

The number of roles an individual plays may decrease with age. A young person, for instance, may be a father, husband, employee, and bridge partner. Old people often identify themselves in only negative or dependent roles, such as widower or social security recipient. The quality of roles changes as social contacts decrease. For example, the father role may persist, but the frequency and quality of contacts with offspring may decrease markedly. The father may feel unwanted or unneeded in this role—a burden rather than a helping and supportive figure. In eliciting the client profile, a discussion of roles helps to determine the person's satisfaction with his or her life.

Information on activity patterns should include data on how an older person spends an average day, in what recreational activities the older person is involved, what he or she enjoys doing, and the degree to which the person is able to carry out activities of daily living (see Chapter 4, Functional Assessment). It is important to determine if the client perceives present behavior as changed or altered from a previous level of functioning, and to note the degree of satisfaction with the current level of functioning. The life space of the individual should be determined and changes assessed. How much is the person able to travel? What resources are available within the neighborhood? Does the older person perceive restrictions within his or her present life space?

The history of activity should be extended to include data on activity patterns during the night and a sleep history. Sleep disturbances are one of the most common complaints of the aged. In general older people tend to report sleeping less at night, having difficulty staying asleep, early awakening, and napping during the daytime. They often have reduced total sleeping time and may have a decrease in deep (Stage 4) sleep. They may report an alteration in patterns of dreaming. The rapid eye movement (REM), or "dream sleep" tends to occur earlier in the sleep cycle and shows an alteration in time interval.

Respiratory, cardiovascular, and metabolic disorders such as diabetes, as well as many medications, interfere with the sleep cycle. Clients experiencing chronic pain, such as occurs with arthritis, experience alterations in the sleep pattern, with multiple and prolonged arousals during the night. A detailed sleep history includes questions to elicit time of retiring, lifelong and current sleep patterns, methods used to facilitate sleep, and perceived effectiveness of sleep.

The older individual's habits in relation to alcohol, tobacco, and caffeine need to be clearly identified because of the significant health risks that are frequently not diagnosed in the elderly and that are associated with the use of these substances. The kind, amount, and frequency per day/week, the emotional and social circumstances associated with use of these substances, and changes in pattern of use over the past year need to be described—as well as any history of desire/efforts to quit their use. The interviewer should note, in particular, any objective signs of alcoholism, such as tremors, breath odor, anger, hostility, and confusion (Starer & Libow, 1990, p. 156).

A complete and detailed nutritional history includes asking what, how much, and how frequently the older individual eats. A typical dietary intake, perhaps including meals eaten over more than one 24-hour interval, should be determined. The adequacy of protein, carbohydrate, fat, fiber, vitamin, mineral, and fluid intake should be noted, as well as the older individual's degree of pleasure in eating, who shops for and prepares the food, the number of hot meals per week, and types of snacks and beverages ingested. Related issues that may be pertinent to explore include the amount of money spent on food (in relation to income and other necessary expenditures), accessibility of stores and kitchen facilities, and any functional limitations in regard to food preparation that may be reversible, for example, visual impairment or limited mobility due to arthritis (Starer & Libow, 1990, p. 156). Further discussion of nutritional assessment and dietary needs of older adults is included in Chapter 8.

Medications are an important cause of symptoms. People over 65 years of age account for only 13% of the U.S. population, but take 25% of the prescription drugs and account for 50% of all adverse drug reactions (Brody et al., 1983). Older adults also take large numbers of over-the-counter drugs. This polypharmacy, in addition to normal age changes and multiple disease conditions, makes the elderly very vulnerable to undesirable drug effects. Studies show that the American population in general is unfamiliar with the name, purpose, and common side effects of medications. Often older people have an added difficulty in knowing their medications due to sensory deficits and the large number of medications taken.

A full history of medications currently being taken, including all prescription, over-the-counter, and home remedies, should be elicited. The client should be urged to bring in the medication bottles for the practitioner to see. Determine how often and at what times during the day each medication is taken, who has prescribed it, how long the client has taken the medication, if the client adjusts or omits dosages for any particular reason, drug expiration dates, and how drugs are stored. The exact dosage of the medication must be clearly documented, as biologic changes that occur with age affect absorption, biotransformation, and excretion of drugs and leave older people at greater risk of developing adverse drug reactions. Medications that commonly cause adverse reactions such as postural hypotension, electrolyte depletion, cognitive dysfunction, or GI bleeding when prescribed for the elderly include antihypertensive drugs, diuretics, digitalis, cimetidine, and nonsteroidal anti-inflammatory agents (NSAIDS).

The practitioner also needs to determine what the client knows about medications, including the purpose and common side effects. During the interview, an effort should be made to identify unsafe practices, such as combining multiple medications in one container or taking drugs prescribed for others. These types of problems can more easily be identified during a home visit. For example, it is not unusual to find that elderly widows still have in their medicine cabinets drugs that were prescribed for their deceased husbands. It is important to ascertain whether the older person is able to read the drug labels and open the containers without difficulty. If family members administer the medicines, they need to be interviewed about how the drugs are given.

Older persons often do not consider over-the-counter items to be medications in the same sense as medically prescribed drugs, although they may have serious side effects and undesirable interactions with prescribed drugs. Therefore, the practitioner often has to elicit data about nonprescription drugs, specifically asking about such items as aspirin, allergy and cold medicines, vitamins, and cathartics. Patterns of abuse of these drugs, as well as noncompliance with prescription drug regimens, can cause serious health problems and will affect decisions about appropriate drug therapy in the future.

Finances are a necessary but often difficult topic to discuss. The older person may feel uneasy revealing that current finances do not cover needs. It is important to keep in mind that inadequate finances affect multiple areas of the elderly person's ability to function. Older people whose finances are minimal or inadequate may be embarrassed to divulge their nutritional intake. For example, an elderly woman was seen in clinic with progressive weakness and edema. Only after a careful history was taken, was it determined that her welfare check was insufficient to buy food for the whole month. The last week of each month she was subsisting on a near starvation diet. As with all topics of a confidential and potentially sensitive nature, approach this in a matter-of-fact way, but with empathy, in order to obtain adequate data.

The sexual history is consistently omitted in health histories of older people. To deny sexuality is to deny a significant aspect of an individual, at any stage in the life cycle. It is now known that the elderly, in both ambulatory and institutional settings, are sexually active into their eighties and nineties. Sexuality implies a broad span of activities and relationships of which sexual intercourse is only one part. The practitioner is concerned with the status of past as well as present loving relationships and the degree to which the client was/is satisfied with these relationships. Even if the person is no longer sexually active, asking questions regarding sexuality shows recognition of the individual, past and present. Widowers and widows need the opportunity to discuss the significance of the loss of a sexual partner.

Interviewing to obtain sexual history can be approached in a variety of ways. It is usually helpful to develop some rapport with the client before asking questions regarding sexuality. Sexuality can be assessed when discussing family relationships or loss of significant others. Physiologic changes that occur with aging may make intercourse and masturbation more difficult. These data can be obtained during the obstetric and gynecologic history when interviewing a woman. For men, obtaining data on the genitourinary system provides a similar opportunity. Ordering data chronologically from adolescence to the present may facilitate data gathering. (See Chapter 9).

Death and dying is another topic frequently avoided in the health history. For older people, death is a reality. It is faced frequently through loss of family and friends. Although older people think about death more frequently, they do not fear death more than younger adults. Many older people can talk easily about the meaning of death. On the other hand, as with many other areas, older people will exhibit cultural and ethnic variations as to their willingness to discuss death. As an example, among some people of Chinese origin discussions of death are seen as a bad omen.

If the practitioner is aware of cues regarding attitudes toward death and separation, the topic can be appropriately inserted into the interview. It may be quite natural for the interviewer to ask about attitudes and feelings toward death when discussing data on availability of and interaction with friends and family or religious practice. When eliciting the client's chief complaint, the practitioner may find that the real concern is fear of a terminal illness and death. Eliciting concerns about adaptation to a chronic disease provides another opportunity to determine attitudes and feelings concerning death.

This may be the logical time to determine if clients have formulated advance directives should they become critically or terminally ill, or should they experience irreversible brain damage. The practitioner should initiate this discussion because, while many older people are eager to discuss advanced planning, they often wait for the practitioner to open the topic. Several documents can help guide a discussion about a values history and advance directives (Gibson, 1990). It is important to determine if a client has expressed verbal wishes and/or has completed written advance directives, that is, treatment directives such as living wills and/or the appointment of a proxy who can act in the person's behalf should he or she become incapacitated (a durable power of attorney for health care). The practitioner may want to have sample documents available that are congruent with state law and that can be shared with the client. It is important to append copies of written directives to the health record, and to determine who else knows about and has copies of written directives.


# FAMILY HISTORY

With the elderly client an elaborate genogram (family tree) may be less meaningful as a predictor of potential health problems, because many familial diseases manifest themselves at an earlier age. Cancer, diabetes, and Alzheimer's disease are exceptions, however. In addition, knowledge of blood relatives (grandparents, aunts, uncles, siblings, children, and spouse) with heart disease, hypertension seizure disorder, mental/emotional disorders, renal and endocrine disease, arthritis, or substance abuse also may indicate physical or psychosocial problems for which the older client and/or the family may be at risk. The family tree of an older individual also still serves as a reference for knowing what past experiences the client has had with diseases, disabilities, and causes of death (Bowers & Thompson, 1988).


# PAST MEDICAL HISTORY

The past medical history is helpful in putting the elderly client's current health problems in perspective. Because the past medical history may be quite lengthy, complicated, and time consuming to amass and organize, it may be helpful to have this portion of the history completed by the client/family at home in advance of the interview. If this information is already available in health records, key points may be confirmed with the older client without needless duplication.

It is important to inquire about allergies and serious illnesses, diseases, and accidents/injuries that may have an impact on the older individual's current health state, including information about diseases and treatments common in the past that are rare today (for example, rheumatic fever and polio). Dates and results of previous health examinations (dental, vision, hearing, proctoscopy, pap smear) as well as Tb skin tests and tetanus, influenza, and pneumovax immunizations, are important since they continue to be recommended preventive services for older adults (U.S. Department of Health & Human Services, 1991). Information about Hepatitis B exposure and immunity status and AIDS testing may be important to ascertain from elders who currently, or in the past, belonged to high risk groups. For this reason it is also important to ascertain whether the older adult has ever received blood transfusions. Data concerning the what, why, when, and where of any surgery, and the older woman's obstetrical history, are also important to obtain. It may be necessary to procure old health records if the older client and family are unable to provide this information (Starer & Libow, 1990, p. 155).

## REVIEW OF SYSTEMS

Guidelines for more specific exploration of the chief complaint(s) and a review of systems (ROS) with elderly clients are included in the subsequent chapters of this book, along with special considerations for each segment of the physical examination. A few general comments are presented in this section to guide the interviewer's approach to obtaining comprehensive, valid, and reliable information in this segment of the health history. There is general consensus among geriatric practitioners that, with the elderly, certain aspects of the history (and physical examination) take precedence over a more typical "head to toe" ROS. Of special concern are the need for a careful review of medications, urinary incontinence, mental status, vision, bowel function, and family and/or other social support (Lavizzo-Mourey, Mezey, & Taylor, 1991, Mezey, Lavizzo-Mourey, Brunswick & Taylor, 1992).

As with younger adults, information concerning the occurrence of symptoms related to the various body systems may be obtained by asking about each listed symptom during the interview. However, it may save time to have the older client who is mentally competent, or a family member, respond to a checklist form prior to the interview. During the interview the nurse can then focus on clarifying and further exploring the symptoms or problem areas that the individual is currently experiencing. Although open-ended questioning is preferable, it is sometimes necessary to ask focused questions and to supply elders with responses from which to choose the one that best describes their symptom/problem. For example, if an elderly male is unable to spontaneously describe the character of his chest pain, it may be useful to ask him to select the best description from a list provided by the interviewer (for example, sharp, dull, stabbing, mild pressure, or crushing).

As with clients of any age, the interviewer should be alert to the likelihood that a "response set" may be operating when review of systems information is gathered. Elders may tend to answer "yes" or "no" indiscriminately to each question on the long list. In particular, be alert to the possibility of common problems that may remain hidden unless specifically asked about; for example, sexual dysfunction, alcohol intake, depression, incontinence, musculoskeletal stiffness, falls, and loss of vision and/or hearing. It is also important to ascertain whether acknowledged, long-standing symptoms have recently changed in quality or in the intensity, duration, or frequency of their occurrence (for example, whether a client currently has to rest three times while climbing a flight of stairs as compared with needing to rest only once during the same activity 2 months ago).

## SUMMARY

To obtain a complete health history from older people requires careful interviewing and data gathering. The practitioner should be aware of factors that affect the communication process between the nurse and older people and should modify the interviewing techniques, setting, and content to meet the special needs of older clients.

## REFERENCES

Bowers, A. C. & Thompson, J. M. (1988). *Clinical manual of health assessment* (pp. 26–27). St. Louis: C.V. Mosby.

Brody, E. M., Kliban, M. H., & Moles, E. (1983). What older people do about their day to day mental and physical health symptoms. *Journal of the American Geriatrics Society, 31,* 489–497.

Burrage, R. L., Dixon, L., & Sehy, Y. (1991). Physical assessment: An overview. In Chenitz, W. C., Stone, J. T., & Salisbury, S. A. (Eds.), *Clinical gerontological nursing: A guide to advanced practice* (pp. 28–29). Philadelphia: Saunders.

Caird, F. I. (1981). Physical examinations of the elderly: Problems and possibilities. In Folmer, A. N. J., & Schontin, J. (Eds.), *Geriatrics for the practitioner. Proceedings of a Seminar held in Amsterdam* (pp. 3–7). Princeton: Exerpta Medica.

——— (1992). *Talking about advance directives: A guide for health care providers.* Choice in Dying, 250 West 57th Street, New York, NY 10107.

Gallo, J. J., Reichel, W. R., & Anderson, L. (1988). *Handbook of geriatric assessment* (pp. 4–8). Gaithersburg, MD: Aspen.

Gibson, J. (1990, Supl.). National values history project. *Generations.* pp. 51–64.

Hale, W.E., Perkins, L.L., May, F.F. et al. (1986). Symptom prevalence in the elderly: An evaluation of age, sex, disease and medication use. *Journal of the American Geriatrics Society, 34*, 333–340.

Lavizzo-Mourey, R., Mezey, M., & Taylor, L. (1991). Completeness of admission of residents assessments in teaching nursing homes. *Journal of the American Geriatrics Society, 39*, 676–682.

Mezey, M., Lavizzo-Mourey, R., Brunswick, J., & Taylor, L. (1992). Consensus among geriatric experts on the components of a complete nursing home admission assessment. *Nurse Practitioner, 17*, 50–61.

Norman, D. C., Grahn, D., & Yoshikawa, T. T. (1985). Fever and aging. *Journal of the American Geriatrics Society, 33*, 859–863.

Peck, R. (1968). Psychological developments in the second half of life. In Neugarten, B. L. (Ed.), *Middle age and aging.* Chicago: University of Chicago Press.

Shanas, E., Townsend, B., Wedderburn, D., et al. (1968). The Psychology of health. In Neugarten, B. L. (Ed.), *Middle age and aging* (p. 215). Chicago: University of Chicago Press.

Starer, P.J., & Libow, L. S. (1990). History and physical examination. In Abrams, W. B. & Berkow, R. (Eds.), *The Merck manual of geriatrics* (pp. 154–156). Rahway, NJ: Merck, Sharp & Dohme.

U.S. Department of Health and Human Services. (1991). *Healthy people 2000: National health promotion and disease prevention.* Rockville, MD: Public Health Service.

*Your Health Care Choices.* Arizona Health Decisions, 122 North Cortez, Suite 210, Prescott, AZ 86301.

## SUGGESTED READINGS

Chenitz, W. C., Stone, J., & Salisbury S. (1991). *Clinical gerontological nursing: A guide to advanced practice.* Philadelphia: W. B. Saunders.

Burke, M., & Walsh M. (1992). *Gerontological nursing: Care of the frail elderly.* St. Louis: Mosby YearBook, Inc.

Eliopoulos, C. (1990). *Health assessment of the older adult.* (2nd ed.). Redwood City, CA: Addison-Wesley Nursing.

Gambert, S. R. (Ed.). (1987). *Handbook of geriatrics.* NY: Plenum Medical Book Co.

Kane, R. L., Ouslander, J. G., & Abrass, I. B. (1989). *Essentials of clinical geriatrics* (2nd ed.). NY: McGraw Hill.

Reichel, W. (1989). *Clinical aspects of aging* (3rd ed.). Philadelphia: Lippincott.

Rossman, I. (1986). *Clinical geriatrics* (3rd ed.). Philadelphia: J.B. Lippincott Co.

Staab, A., & Lyles, M. (1990). *Manual of geriatric nursing.* Glenville, IL: Scott Foresman/Little Brown.

Stokes, S. A., Rauckhorst, L., & Mezey, M. (1975). *Physical assessment of the aged person.* Spring Valley, NY: Blue Hill Education Systems, Inc.

# 4

# Functional Assessment

Function is one of, if not the, most important components of health for older people. With increasing age, chronic illnesses and commonly occurring age changes often impair function and threaten independence. Close to 50% of people 65 and over, and 60% of people 85 and over have some degree of limitation of daily activities (NIA Conference on Assessment, 1983). Because preserving activity is a key health objective, determining function is integral to the health assessment of the elderly.

Functional assessment can serve multiple purposes: to describe group differences; to assist family decision making; to determine level of care and reimbursement; to enhance diagnosis and management in clinical practice; and for research. Here we discuss the application of functional assessment to clinical practice and define functional assessment in the narrow sense of ability to function in everyday life.

So defined, functional assessment usually involves two components: 1) activities of daily living (ADL), which reflect people's ability to manage their personal care; and 2) instrumental activities of daily living (IADL), which reflect people's ability to live independently in the community. As such, functional assessment is only one of many domains of comprehensive geriatric assessment. Psychosocial and mental health assessment, which obviously impact on function, are discussed in Chapters 13 and 11, respectively. Musculoskeletal assessment is discussed in Chapter 10.

Clinical data about a person's ability to function can be obtained during the normal course of a history and physical examination or through the use of standardized paper and pencil or performance-based functional assessment instruments. This chapter identifies several commonly used standardized measures of functional assessment and discusses the advantages and disadvantages of systematic functional assessment in comparison to assessing function solely within the traditional history and physical examination. A more complete resource for functional assessment instruments appears in the Bibliography at the end of the chapter. Developing a file of commonly used functional assessment instruments can help the practitioner tailor the assessment to the client's health and functional status.

## HISTORY OF FUNCTIONAL ASSESSMENT

In geriatrics most practitioners determine a history of functional capacity by using a combination of standardized instruments and a detailed history. Standardized instruments provide valid and reliable data about an older persons's self-perception of his or her functional ability. This information is completed by the patients themselves, for example, in the waiting room prior to the visit, or ascertained during the course of the patient history. Responses on the assessment instrument serve as a springboard for a more detailed exploration of functional ability between the patient and provider.

## Measures of Activities of Daily Living (ADL)

Measures of ADL reflect people's ability to perform tasks of basic personal care: eating, ambulating, transferring, dressing, bathing, toileting, and continence. As with all assessment instruments, the purpose is of primary importance when selecting ADL instruments. The Katz scale, for example, uses only dichotomous ratings of independent/dependent (Kane & Kane, 1988). Other scales provide a greater differentiation between levels of performance and need for assistance. The Lawton Scale (Table 4.1) is probably the most commonly used ADL scale and differentiates based on need for personal assistance (Lawton, 1971). Other instruments, for example the Barthel Self Care Rating, further differentiate between whether an activity is performed totally independently, with human aid, or use of an assistive device, and whether the activity is performed in a reasonable amount of time (Kane & Kane, 1988). Some scales differentiate even further to reflect frequency of performance, that is daily, several times a day, etc.

## TABLE 4.1 Physical Self-maintenance Scale (ADL)*

Toilet
1. Cares for self at toilet completely; no incontinence.
2. Needs to be reminded, or needs help in cleaning self, or has rare (weekly at most) accidents.
3. Soiling or wetting while asleep, more than once a week.
4. No control of bowels or bladder.

Feeding
1. Eats without assistance.
2. Eats with minor assistance at meal times, with help in preparing food, or with help in cleaning up after meals.
3. Feeds self with moderate assistance and is untidy.
4. Needs major assistance in feeding but cooperates with efforts of others to help.
5. Completely unable to feed self and resists efforts of others to help.

Dressing
1. Dresses, undresses, and selects clothes from own wardrobe.
2. Dresses and undresses self, with minor assistance.
3. Needs moderate assistance in dressing or selection of clothes.
4. Needs major assistance in dressing but cooperates with efforts of others to help.
5. Completely unable to dress self and resists efforts of others to help.

Grooming (neatness, hair, nails, hands, face, clothing)
1. Always neatly dressed and well-groomed, without assistance.
2. Grooms self adequately, with occasional minor assistance (e.g., in shaving)
3. Needs moderate and regular assistance or supervision in grooming.
4. Needs total grooming care, but can remain well-groomed after help from others.
5. Actively negates all efforts of others to maintain grooming.

Physical Ambulation
1. Goes about grounds or city.
2. Ambulates within residence or about one block distance.
3. Ambulates with assistance of (check one):

    ☐ wheelchair  ☐ railing      ☐ cane, or  ☐ walker;
    1. ☐ gets in and out without help;    2. ☐ needs help in getting in and out

4. Sits unsupported in chair or wheelchair, but cannot propel self without help.
5. Bedridden more than half the time.

Bathing
1. Bathes self (tub, shower, sponge bath) without help.
2. Bathes self, with help in getting in and out of tub.
3. Washes face and hands only, but cannot bathe rest of body.
4. Does not wash self, but is cooperative with those who bathe him/her.
5. Does not try to wash self, and resists efforts to keep clean.

*Start by asking the patient to describe her/his ability to perform a given activity, e.g., feeding. Then ask specific questions as needed.

Reprinted with permission of the American Geriatrics Society. "The Functional Assessment of Elderly People," by M.P. Lawton, *Journal of the American Geriatrics Society, 9*(6), pp. 465–481, 1971.

## Measures of Instrumental Activities of Daily Living (IADL)

IADL refers to activities more complex than those needed for ADL and associated with living independently in the community: cooking, cleaning, laundry, shopping, using the telephone, transportation, and managing finances. As with ADL scales, IADL scales differ as to their comprehensiveness. Some take into account sex variations in performance of IADL activities; others reflect frequency of performance; still others control for perceptual or memory deficits which may influence performance.

The Lawton IADL Scale, a commonly used IADL measure, is shown in Table 4.2. This IADL scale differentiates as to whether the activity is performed with no, minimal, or substantial assistance, or not at all (Lawton, 1971).

The very old, women, poor, and minority clients exhibit the greatest dependency in ADL and IADL. For example, only 7% of white middle-class males aged 65 and over have IADL deficits, in contrast to 28% of older non-white females living in communities with >15% of people below the poverty line (Jette, Branch, & Berlin, 1991).

There is moderate evidence of a hierarchy of needs related to functional performance. For example, people who can eat independently are also independent in dressing. Ability to cut one's own toenails has been shown to correlate strongly with full independence in ADL (Townsend & Shamas, 1968). Independence in IADL does not, however, necessarily imply full independence in ADL. People may be totally independent in IADL, for example, and still be incontinent or unable to bathe in a bathtub independently. Impairment of fine motor coordination of the hands and wrist is associated with ADL deficits, while IADL function is more commonly impaired as a result of lower extremity decrements (Elston, Koch, & Weissert, 1991).

## Objective, Performance Based Measures of Functional Assessment

Most geriatric practitioners begin their observations as to a persons functional status by watching people walk into the examining room, sit down and stand up from a chair, undress and dress, and climb onto the examining table. Some practitioners add procedures to test fine motor coordination, such as buttoning clothes and opening doors. When concerned about continence, practitioners may also observe patients as they use the toilet. The musculoskeletal and neurological examination add additional information, especially about muscle

**TABLE 4.2 Scale for Instrumental Activities of Daily Living (IADL)***

Ability to Telephone
  1. Operates telephone on own initiative: looks up and dials numbers, etc.
  2. Dials a few well-known numbers.
  3. Answers telephone but does not dial.
  4. Does not use telephone at all.

Shopping
  1. Takes care of all shopping needs independently.
  2. Shops independently for small purchases.
  3. Needs to be accompanied on any shopping trip.
  4. Completely unable to shop.

Food Preparation
  1. Plans, prepares, and serves adequate meals independently.
  2. Prepares adequate meals if supplied with ingredients.
  3. Heats and serves prepared meals, or prepares meals but does not maintain adequate diet.
  4. Needs to have meals prepared and served.

Housekeeping
  1. Maintains house alone or with occasional assistance (e.g., heavy work done by domestic help).
  2. Performs light daily tasks such as dishwashing and bedmaking.
  3. Performs light daily tasks but cannot maintain acceptable level of cleanliness.
  4. Needs help with all home maintenance tasks.
  5. Does not participate in any housekeeping tasks.

Laundry
  1. Does personal laundry completely.
  2. Launders small items: rinses socks, stockings, etc.
  3. All laundry must be done by others.

Mode of Transportation
  1. Travels independently on public transportation or drives own car.
  2. Arranges own travel via taxi but does not otherwise use public transportation.
  3. Travels on public transportation when assisted or accompanied by another.
  4. Travels limited to taxi or automobile, with assistance of another.
  5. Does not travel at all.

Responsibility for Own Medication
  1. Is responsible for taking medication in correct dosages at correct time.
  2. Takes responsibility if medication is prepared in advance in separate dosages.
  3. Is not capable of dispensing own medication.

Ability to Handle Finances
  1. Manages financial matters independently (budgets, writes checks, pays rent and bills, goes to bank); collects and keeps track of income.
  2. Manages day-to-day purchases but needs help with banking, major purchases, etc.
  3. Incapable of handling money.

*Start by asking the patient to describe her/his functioning in each category; then complement with specific questions as needed.

Reprinted with permission of the American Geriatrics Society. "The Functional Assessment of Elderly People" by M.P. Lawton, *Journal of the American Geriatrics Society*, 9(6), pp. 465–481, 1971.

strength, joint mobility, overall stability (the Romberg test) and position and vibratory sensation. (See also Chapters 10 and 12). Thus, a typical patient encounter and physical examination yields a rather comprehensive picture of a person's functional ability.

Systematic performance-based measurement of functional status is relatively new. While many of the early functional assessment instruments were designed as performance-based measures, concern for identifying people at risk for falling has spurred a resurgence of interest in direct measurement of functional capacity. Several direct measures of function have been developed which can readily be adapted for use in clinical practice. One such measure, the Structured Assessment & Independent Living Skills (SAILS) is shown in Table 4.3 (Mahurin, Debettignies, & Pirozzola, 1991). For a more complete discussion of performance measures in musculoskeletal and falls assessment, see Chapter 10.

**TABLE 4.3 Structured Assessment of Independent Living Skills (SAILS): Scoring Form**

| Scoring form | | | | |
|---|---|---|---|---|
| Name: | | | | Date: |
| Age: | Sex: | Handedness: | Education: | Examiner: |
| Diagnosis: | | | | |

Note: If patient is unable to complete task, assign maximum time of 60" unless otherwise indicated

*MOTOR TASKS*

| *Fine Motor skills* | Time | Score |
|---|---|---|
| 1. Picks up coins<br>      0 = drops two   1 = drops one<br>      2 = slow   3 = normal (8")<br>2. Removes wrappers<br>      0 = needs assistance    1 = tears one or more<br>      2 = slow     3 = normal   (35")<br>3. Cuts with scissors<br>      0 = can't cut   1 = off line  2 = slow  3 = normal   (32")<br>4. Folds letter and places in envelope<br>      0 = can't fold   1 = doesn't fit   2 = slow<br>      3 = normal  (16")<br>5. Uses key in lock<br>      0 = can't insert   1 = can't unlock   2 = slow<br>      3 = normal  (13") | | |
| Subtotal: | | |

| *Gross Motor Skills* | Time | Score |
|---|---|---|
| 1. Stands up from sitting<br>      0 = unable   1 = uses arms of chair   2 = slow<br>      3 = normal  (2") | | |

*(continued)*

**TABLE 4.3 (*continued*)**

2. Opens and walks through
        0 = unable    1 = needs door held open    2 = slow
        3 = normal   (5")
3. Regular gait
        0 = unable    1 – assistive device    2 = slow
        3 = normal   (6")
Time 1)____ 2)____ Mean____ Steps 1)____ 2)____ Mean____
4. Tandem gait
        0 = unable, steps off 4 or more times
        1 = steps off 2–3 times    2 = slow (1 step allowed)
        3 = normal   (9")
Time 1)____ 2)____ Mean____ Steps off line 1)____ 2)____ Mean____
5. Transfers object across room
        0 = drops    1 = inaccurate placement
        2 = slow   3 = normal
Time 1)____ 2)____ Mean____

Subtotal:

| *Dressing Skills* | Time | Score |
|---|---|---|

1. Puts on shirt (max. = 102")
        0 = can't put on or button    1 = misaligned
        2 = slow   3 = normal   (86")
2. Buttons cuffs of shirt
        0 = unable    1 = one cuff    2 = slow
        3 = normal   (45")
3. Puts on jacket
        0 = can't put on    1 = needs help with zipper
        2 = slow   3 = normal   (27")
4. Ties shoelaces
        0 = unable/wrong feet    1 = knot comes undone
        2 = slow   3 = normal   (9")
5. Puts on gloves
        0 = unable    1 = one hand   2 = slow   3 = normal (21")

Subtotal:

| *Eating Skills* | Time | Score |
|---|---|---|

1. Drinks from glass
        0 = unable    1 = spills    2 = slow    3 = normal   (3")
2. Transfers food with spoon
        0 = unable    1 = drops    2 = slow    3 = normal   (11")
3. Cuts with fork and knife
        0 = unable    1 = drops    2 = slow    3 = normal   (16")
4. Transfers food with fork
        0 = unable    1 = drops    2 = slow    3 = normal   (16")
5. Transfers liquid with spoon
        0 = unable    1 = spills    2 = slow    3 = normal   (13")

Subtotal:

Total Motor Time_____     Total Motor Score_____

**COGNITIVE TASKS**

**Expressive Language**                                 Score

(*continued*)

**TABLE 4.3** (*continued*)

Scoring form

Name:                                                                    Date:

Age:    Sex:    Handedness:    Education:    Examiner:

Diagnosis:

---

1. Quality of expression
   0 = severe <25%    1 = moderate 25–90%
   2 = mild 90–99%    3 = intact
2. Repetition
   0 = no items    1 = 1 item    2 = 2 items    3 = all 3 items
3. Object naming
   0 = 3 or less    1 = 4 items    2 = 5 items    3 = all 6 items
4. Writes legible note
   0 = illegible    1 = 1 item    2 = 2 items    3 = all 3 items
5. Completes application form
   0 = 3 or less    1 = 4 items    2 = 5 items    3 = all 6 items

Subtotal:

*Receptive Language*                                                      Score

1. Reads and follows printed instructions
   0 = none    1 = 1 item    2 = 2 items    3 = all 3 items
2. Understands written material
   0 = none    1 = 1–4 items    2 = 5 items    3 = all 6 items
   Article 1: Correct 1)____    2)____    3)____
   Article 2: Correct 1)____    2)____    3)____
3. Understands common signs
   0 = none    1 = 1 item    2 = 2 items    3 = all 3 items
4. Follows verbal directions
   0 = none    1 = 1 item    2 = 2 items    3 = all 3 items
   1) Touch shoulder    2) Hands on table, close eyes
   3) Draw circle, hand pencil, fold paper
5. Identifies named objects
   0 = none    1 = 1 item    2 = 2 items    3 = all 3 items

Subtotal:

*Time Orientation*                                                        Score

1. States time on clock (6:14)
   0 = off over 1 hour    1 = off within 1 hour
   2 = off 10 minutes    3 = correct within 1 minute
2. Calculates time interval (until 7:30)
   0 = off 1 hour    1 = off within 1 hour
   2 = off within 15 minutes    3 = correct within 1 minute
3. States time of alarm setting (8:15)
   0 = off 1 hour    1 = off within 1 hour
   2 = off within 15 minutes    3 = correct within 1 minute
4. Locates current date on calendar
   0 = incorrect month    1 = correct month
   2 = correct week    3 = correct date
5. Correctly reads calendar
   0 = none    1 = 1 item    2 = 2 items    3 = all 3 items
   1) Fridays    2) Day of 15th    3) 2nd Monday

Subtotal:

(*continued*)

**TABLE 4.3** (*continued*)

| *Money-Related Skills* | Score |
|---|---|

1. Counts money
      0 = none   1 = 1 item   2 = 2 items   3 = all 3 items
      1) 35 cents_____   2) 95 cents_____   3) $1.41_____
2. Makes change
      0 = none   1 = 1 item   2 = 2 items   3 = all 3 items
      1) ($.75 from $1.00) = $.25____
      2) ($.41 from $.50) = $.09____
      3) ($2.79 from $5.00) = $2.21____
3. Understands monthly utility bill
      0 = none   1 = 1 item   2 = 2 items   3 = all 3 items
      1) (Light Co.)____   2) ($38.46)____   3) (3/6/87)____
4. Writes check
      0 = 2 or less   1 = 3 items   2 = 4 items   3 = all 5 items
      1) Date  2) Payee  3) Numerical amount
      4) Written amount  5) Signature
5. Understands checkbook
      0 = none   1 = 1 item   2 = 2 items   3 = all 3 items
      1) Checks on August 11  2) Check #355
      3) Balance ($440.40)

Subtotal: _____

Total Cognitive Score _____

| *Instrumental Activities* | Score |
|---|---|

1. Uses telephone book
      0 = none   1 = 1 item   2 = 2 items   3 = all 3 items
2. Dials telephone number
      0 = cannot handle phone   1 = misdials number
      2 = needs help to read   3 = correctly reads and dials
3. Understands medication label
      0 = none   1 = 1 item   2 = 2 items   3 = all 3 items
4. Opens medication container
      0 = can't open two   1 = can't open one
      2 = needs cue   3 = normal
5. Follows simple recipe
      0 = unable   1 = 1 step   2 = 2 steps   3 = all 3 steps

Subtotal: _____

| *Social Interaction* | Score |
|---|---|

1. Responds to greeting and farewell
      0 = none   1 = 1 item   2 = 2 items   3 = all 3 items
2. Responds to request for information
      0 = none   1 = 1 item   2 = 2 items   3 = all 3 items
3. Responds to social directives
      0 = none   1 = 1 item   2 = 2 items   3 = all 3 items
4. Requests needed information
      0 = none   1 = 1 item   2 = 2 items   3 = all 3 items
5. Understands non-verbal expression
      0 = none   1 = 1 item   2 = 2 items   3 = all 3 items

Subtotal: _____

GRAND TOTAL SCORE_____

*Note.* From "Structured Assessment of Independent Living Skills: Preliminary Report of a Performance Measure of Functional Abilities in Dementia," by R. Mahurin, B. Debettignies, and F. Pirozzola, 1991, *Journal of Gerontology, 46*, pp. 58–66. Reprinted with permission. Copyright © The Gerontological Society of America.

## Advantages and Disadvantages of the use of Standardized Functional Assessment Instruments

The benefits of using standardized functional assessment instruments are shown in Table 4.4. The major benefits accrue from focusing provider questions on those aspects of the history of greatest concern to patients, and on identifying what patients realistically can and wish to be able to do. Functional assessment has proven useful in identifying previously undiagnosed and often highly treatable conditions and in improving diagnostic and therapeutic outcomes. By tracking change in function over time, providers can potentially identify reversible causes of deficits or early evidence of disease.

Because functional assessment provides a framework in which to evaluate the consequences of chronic illness from the patient's perspective, it broadens the data base on which to make treatment decisions and assists patients and providers in choosing the degree to which certain diseases should be treated.

Standardized instruments have the advantage of assuring that all practitioners who see the patient at different encounters ask a uniform set of questions to determine function. Ascribed functional levels can easily be incorporated into a flow sheet so as to be monitored over time. Such data focuses the efforts of different health disciplines on common patient goals and evaluation of treatment effectiveness, and can be reliably reassessed in different settings.

A further advantage of standardized instruments is that they require little time to administer. Most ADL and IADL scales can be completed

---

**TABLE 4.4 Advantages of Functional Assessment Instruments**

Focuses the encounter on what patients can and wish to do.
Elicits data of greatest concern to patients.
Standardizes the functional history.
Yields consistent data collected by same professional over time and by different
    professionals who see the patient.
Provides objective data for use in flow sheet.
Yields quantifiable data on which to base and evaluate therapeutic recommen-
    dations to patients and families.
Identifies potentially reversible functional deficits.
Improves diagnosis and treatment.
Focuses health care team on uniform outcome goals.
Broadens data base on which to make decisions regarding resource utilization,
    referrals, and placement.
Provides benchmark for decisions to use or withhold treatment.
Objective data which can move across health care settings.

in less than 5 minutes, giving the practitioner a "snapshot" of a person's ability to maneuver in the environment.

Practitioners should recognize, however, that functional assessment instruments have certain drawbacks which limit their usefulness in clinical practice. These limitations are listed in Table 4.5.

Most instruments yield little or no information as to the frequency with which an activity is performed, the time required to complete the activity, or the reasons why an activity is not being performed. Moreover, most instruments assume that every activity is of equal importance, whereas patients are more likely to ascribe greater importance to some activities and lower or no importance to others; overall composite scores, therefore, may yield an inaccurate picture of the person's true functional status.

Most practitioners believe that functional status is most accurately assessed by direct observation in the person's own home. Self-report instruments, while yielding remarkably accurate information, depict only the person's current level of function rather than actual or potential functional capacity. Such instruments may not reflect the patient's best possible or even typical function, and are subject to the influence of mood and memory.

The use of performance-based tests, on the other hand, is also not without risk. Performance in the office or clinic, which is an artificial setting, may not reflect people's "typical" performance in their home environment. Older people may feel embarrassed or self-conscious about demonstrating skills in front of a health care provider. Evaluation in the person's home, while much preferred to office assessment, still poses problems as to time and expense. Moreover, irrespective of whether it is in the person's home or not, one observation is rarely sufficient to capture a comprehensive picture of the person's performance level.

It is important to emphasize that most instruments fail to capture the range of activities of very active adults or the small changes in

**TABLE 4.5 Disadvantages of Functional Assessment Instruments**

Do not reflect reasons why an activity is not performed, frequency of performance, or relative importance of activities.
Capture neither the range of activities of very active adults or small changes in activity.
Fail to address people's fears about revealing functional deficits.
Do not show how people actually function in the "real world."
Measure actual function rather than performance capacity.
Are subject to errors of recall and mood.

activities expected, for example, during a rehabilitation program. For very active older adults, most of the questions on an ADL scale would be superfluous. On the other hand, for assessing improvements following a cerebral vascular accident, measures of ADL and IADL are far too gross. The practitioner would do better to use range of motion inventories or the more detailed self-care evaluation measures, examples of which are mentioned in the references at the end of this chapter.

Lastly, it is important to keep in mind that functional assessment instruments are *not* comprehensive measures of health assessment (Table 4.6). Self-report instruments have few or no questions, for example, concerning the use of functional aides such as walkers or canes. They fail to assess risk for injury, rest and sleep pattern, sensory deficits, or aspects of medication use which may markedly influence function. It is therefore important to use standardized instruments in conjunction with, rather than as a substitute for, a comprehensive history and physical examination.

Consequently, most practitioners choose to supplement information gained from standardized instruments with a more detailed history of function. For example, hearing that an older person has continued to drive a car leads to a myriad of questions: does the person drive long distances? at night? are there any problems with glare? are reflexes good? any near misses? any accidents? is the person comfortable driving?

In questioning the client it is essential to include questions regarding recreational activities, changes between past and present activity levels, the variety of current physical activities, as well as expectations and level of satisfaction with what the older client is able to do. Fears of decreasing capabilities and the effect that they may have on the client's present functional level should be elicited. If the client is experiencing limitations in activity, it is important to ascertain whether these

**TABLE 4.6 Aspects of a Health Assessment Not Included in Most Functional Assessment Instruments**

Use of functional aides
Leisure activities
Rest and sleep pattern
Incontinence
Injury potential
Nutrition
Medication use
Impaired cognition/stress/depression
Sensory changes
Functional changes associated with specific diseases

are due to physical, financial, or social factors outside of the older person's control, or whether they are predominantly self-imposed due to fear or social withdrawal.

At subsequent visits, past and present performances are compared and explanations for changes explored. Change in activity may occur not only from deterioration in health but also because of lack of interest or motivation. In other instances, function may be maintained but with greater effort or less pleasure.

## Recommendations for Obtaining a Functional Assessment

General recommendations as to when to perform a systematic functional assessment are shown in Table 4.7. Function should be assessed routinely as part of an initial and annual visit for all people 65 and over. On admission to a nursing home, functional assessment should be completed within the first week of admission. On subsequent encounters, the practitioner should determine whether the patient's function has improved, worsened, or is unchanged since the previous visit.

Functional status should be reassessed whenever a patient's health status changes, for example, subsequent to hospitalization, nursing home or rehabilitation facility placement, after an episode of acute illness or exacerbation of a chronic illness, and during the rehabilitation phase following functional decline. Reassessment provides a comparison with past performance and objective evidence of improvement, stabilization, or decline.

A record of the most recent functional assessment should accompany patients when they enter a new health care facility. This helps new providers formulate both a realistic picture of the person's most recent performance, and helps to establish appropriate goals for therapy.

**TABLE 4.7 When to Perform a Systematic Functional Assessment**

Routinely as part of an initial and annual visit for all people 65 and over.
When patient's status changes, for example subsequent to:
      hospitalization
      nursing home or rehabilitation placement
      an acute illness
      exacerbation of a chronic illness
At set intervals for populations "ar risk," for example, patients with:
      Parkinson's disease
      frequent falls
      severe arthritis

It should be recognized that place, timing, and perceived purpose for eliciting information may markedly influence functional assessment data. Older people who live in the community are aware that functional deficits may limit their ability to live independently. Institutionalized elders recognize that further functional declines may cause them to be transferred to another unit. Thus people may perceive reasons for minimizing or maximizing functional deficits unless the purpose for eliciting the data is clearly explained and the provider maintains a nonjudgmental attitude when eliciting information.

## REFERENCES

Elston, J., Koch, G., & Weissert, W. (1991). Regression-adjusted small area estimates of functional dependence in the noninstitutionalized American population age 65 and over. *American Journal of Public Health, 81*, 335–43.

Jette, A., Branch, L., & Berlin, J. (1991). Musculoskeletal impairments and physical disablement among the aged. *The Journals of Gerontology, 45*, M203–208.

Kane, R. A., & Kane, R. L. (1988). *Assessing the elderly: A practical guide to measurement.* Lexington MA: Lexington Books.

Lawton, M. P. (1971). The functional assessment of elderly people. *Journal of the American Geriatrics Society, 9*(6), 465–481.

Mahurin, R., Debettignies, B., & Pirozzola, F. (1991). Structured assessment of independent living skills: Preliminary report of a performance measure of functional abilities in dementia. *Journal of Gerontology, 46*, 258–66.

NIA Conference on Assessment. (1983). *Journal of the American Geriatrics Society, 31*(11) & *31*(12), 636–765.

Townsend, P., Shanas, E. (1968). The psychology of health. In Neugarten, B. (Ed.), *Middle age and aging: A reader in social psychology.* Chicago: The University of Chicago Press.

## SUGGESTED READINGS

Almy, T. (1988). Comprehensive functional assessment for elderly patients (position paper). *Annals of Internal Medicine, 109*(7), 70–72.

Applegate, W. B., Blass, J., & Franklin, T. (1990). Instruments for the functional assessment of older patients. *The New England Journal of Medicine, 322*, 1207–1214.

Benoliel, I., McCorkle, R., & Young, K. (1980). Development of a social dependency scale. *Research in Nursing and Health, 3*, 3–10.

Burke, M., & Walsh, M. (1992). *Gerontological nursing: Care of the frail elderly.* St. Louis: Mosby Yearbook, Inc.

Chenitz, W. C., Stone, J., & Salisbury, S. (1991). *Clinical gerontological nursing: A guide to advanced practice*. Philadelphia: W. B. Saunders.

Eliopoulos, C. (1990). *Health assessment of the older adult* (2nd ed.). Redwood City, CA: Addison-Wesley Nursing.

Fillenbaum, C. (1985). Screening the elderly: A brief instrumental activities of daily living measure. *Journal of the American Geriatrics Society, 33*, 698–706.

Fulton, J., Katz, S., Jack, S., & Hendershot, G. (1989, March). Physical functioning of the aged. *Vital and Health Statistics*, Series 10, No. 107. Hyattsville, MD: National Center for Health Statistics.

Johnson, J., & Mezey, M. (1990). Functional status assessment: An approach to tertiary care. In Lavizzo-Mourey, R., Day, S., Diserens, D., & Grisso, J. A. (Eds.) *Practicing prevention for the elderly*. Philadelphia: Hanley & Belfus.

Lawton, M. P. (1988). Scales to measure competence in everyday activities. *Psychopharmacology Bulletin, 24*, 609–614.

Lueckenotte, A. (1990). *Pocket Guide to Gerontologic Assessment*. St. Louis: Mosby Yearbook, Inc.

National Institute of Health. (1988). National Institute of Health consensus development conference statement: Geriatric assessment methods for clinical decision making. *Journal of the American Geriatrics Society, 36*, 342–347.

Rubenstein, L., Calkins, D., Greenfield et al. (1989). Health status assessment for elderly patients. Report of the Society of General Internal Medicine task force on health assessment. *Journal of the American Geriatric Society, 37*, 562–569.

Rubenstein, L., & Wieland, D. (1989). Comprehensive geriatric assessment. In Lawton, P. (Ed.) *Annual Review of Gerontology and Geriatrics*, Volume 9, 145–196.

Tinetti, M., & Ginter, S. (1988). Identifying mobility dysfunctions in elderly patients. *Journal of the American Medical Association, 259*, 1190–1193.

Tinetti, M., Speechley, M., & Ginter, S. (1988). Risk factors for falls among elderly persons living in the community. *New England Journal of Medicine, 319*, 1701–1707.

Williams, M., Hadler, N., & Earp, J. (1982). Manual ability as a marker of dependency in geriatric women. *Journal of Chronic Disease, 35*, 115–122.

# Assessment of General Appearance, Skin, Hair, Feet, Nails, and Endocrine Status

## HISTORY

### Client Profile

In beginning to gather data about general appearance and skin, the nurse should elicit how the older person feels about him or herself and determine if there are any perceived changes in general appearance. It is preferable to let the client spontaneously tell about changes that have been noted and then the practitioner can ask specific questions concerning any height, weight, or tissue distribution changes to complete the data base. Has the client noted any loss in stature? Do clothes fit differently—are they longer or tighter? Have alterations been necessary? It is especially important to ascertain the level of the client's comfort or discomfort with changes in appearance. For example, when comparing themselves to other older persons, clients may express positive feelings about themselves by such statements as, "I don't shuffle my feet."

## Past Health History

Significant past health history about the skin includes exposure of the skin to the sun and the use of protective skin products. Fair people with high sun exposure, especially in childhood, are at increased risk for skin cancer. The client's patterns of medication use may also provide important data related to the occurrence of skin eruptions, especially since older people tend to take multiple medications. Allergies to medication or susceptibility to skin eruptions in the past should also be ascertained. A past history of irradiation to the skin alerts the practitioner to the potential for localized and also for systemic lesions, such as hypothyroidism resulting from past irradiation to the head or neck.

## Review of Systems

### Skin

Data about the skin should begin with patterns of self-care including frequency of bathing and use of products such as alcohol and sun blocks. The history may elicit perceived changes in texture, color, elasticity, thickness, and loss of subcutaneous tissue. The older client may have noted wrinkling, decreased sweating, itching, and increased sensitivity to cold. Patterns of self-care of the skin help to ascertain whether symptoms such as pruritus and/or dryness of the skin are secondary to normal age changes, to inappropriate methods of skin care, or to pathologic conditions such as diabetes mellitus.

A history of exposure to sunlight is relevant to assessing the older client's risk of skin cancer. As at any age, a history of a sore that has not healed, or a mole that has changed in size, shape, or color should be further investigated. The practitioner should obtain a history of iatrogenically induced skin lesions. Antibiotics and barbiturates frequently cause skin rashes in the aged. Specific questions regarding skin lesions that are more common in older clients are suggested in the physical examination section on skin.

Evidence of bruising or skin abrasions should alert the practitioner to the possibility of elder abuse. Several instruments are available to assist the practitioner evaluate the potential for mistreatment in the elderly (Fulmer, 1989).

### Hair

When the older client reports changes in the texture, color, amount, or distribution of body, facial, or scalp hair, it is important to assess whether these changes are characteristic of normal aging or due to disease. Scalp dryness is a normal and common complaint. The post-menopausal woman may report distress due to the development of chin whiskers secondary to hormonal changes. Men can be questioned as to their past and current use, success with, and side effects associated with the topical application of minoxidil (Rogaine) to combat baldness (Kuhn, 1991).

## Feet and Nails

It is estimated that 80% of older people report some problems with their feet and nails (Schank, 1977). Questions should determine the specific method of foot hygiene used by the client and presence of the most commonly reported foot problems. The incidence of foot problems commonly occurring in older people is presented in Table 5.1. History data should further delineate the shoe fit and any change in size or type of shoe worn. Restrictions in activities of daily living attributed to foot problems should be noted.

Information about common alterations in the nails, such as thickening and color changes, may be elicited during the history. The practitioner should assess the adequacy of the older client's pattern of nail care. Does the client see a podiatrist, trim his or her own finger and toenails, or have a friend or relative who is available to provide this service? If the client trims his or her own nails, does the client have the necessary coordination and expertise to do it safely?

**TABLE 5.1 Incidence of Foot Problems in a Group of Older Persons (n = 377)**

| Problem | N | Incidence (%) |
| --- | --- | --- |
| Calluses | 169 | 45 |
| Bunions | 155 | 41 |
| Toenail problems | 137 | 36 |
|   Mycotic nails | 32 | 8 |
|   Ingrown nails | 82 | 22 |
|   Hypertrophied nails | 23 | 6 |
| Corns | 132 | 35 |
| Fungus infections | 91 | 24 |
| Hammer toes | 53 | 14 |
| Edema | 37 | 10 |
| Circulatory problems | 29 | 8 |
| Bacterial infections | 3 | 1 |
| Dermatitis | 6 | 2 |

Note. Adapted from "Foot Education and Screening Programs for the Elderly," by D. Conrad, 1977, Journal of Gerontological Nursing, 3(6), p. 15.

*Endocrine*

Symptoms of endocrine disorders will be the same in the older client as at any age, except for hyperthyroidism. This disorder in the older client is more likely to manifest itself with symptoms of apathy, depression, and emaciation, rather than hyperkinesia and restlessness. Atrial fibrillation may be the most helpful indication of thyroid hyperactivity. Myxedema (hypothyroidism) is the most common thyroid disorder in advanced age and, although its overall frequency is not increased in the older age group, its symptoms are often misdiagnosed and attributed to "old age," atherosclerosis, vitamin deficiencies, or anemia. Because the incidence of diabetes mellitus is increased in the older population, it is essential to explore fully the appropriate questions in the review of systems regarding weight loss, appetite changes, thirst, and polyuria.

## PHYSICAL EXAMINATION

## General Appearance

Physical examination begins with observation of general appearance. Older people demonstrate a generalized decrease in stature, ranging from 6 to 10 cm from onset of maturity to old age. While the longer bones do not undergo changes, osteoporosis produces a decrease in the size of smaller, trabecular bones. The shoulder width is decreased and flexion occurs at the knees and hips. A narrowing of the intervertebral discs causes diminished size of the intervertebral and intercostal spaces (see Figure 5.1).

Senile kyphosis (dowager's or widow's hump), an increased curvature of the thoracic spine, occurs commonly. In an attempt to compensate for this deformity, there is a backward tilting of the head and a shortening of the neck, causing the lateral view of the head, neck, and thorax to resemble a rounded E. These age changes also result in the arm span being greater than the height and contribute to the gangly appearance often seen in older people.

Additional age changes contribute to the characteristic physical appearance of older people. The total number of body cells diminishes and accounts for evident connective tissue changes. There is a decrease in the amount and elasticity of subcutaneous tissue. Muscle bulk, mass, and tone are lost, and there is a decrease and redistribution of the total body fat. There is a sharpening of the contours and deepening of the hollows of the body. This is especially apparent around the orbits of the eyes, the supraclavicular fossa, the intercostal spaces, and pelvis.

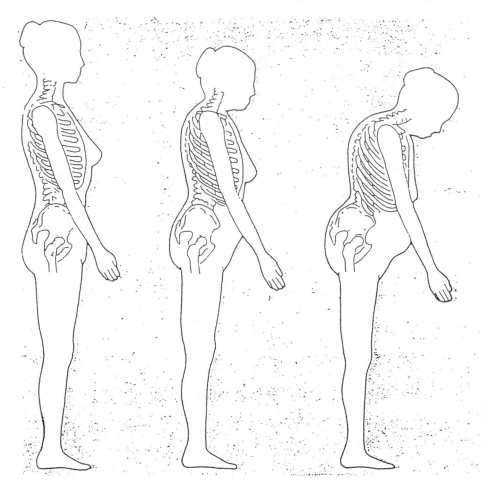

**FIGURE 5.1 Posture changes commonly seen in older people. As osteoporosis weakens bones, fractures of vertebrae cause women to become stooped from the waist up, with a height loss of four inches or more.**

Reprinted with permission from *Stand Tall! The Informed Woman's Guide to Preventing Osteoporosis* by Morris Notelovits and Marsha Ware, 1982, Triad Publishing Co.

The body takes on a bony or angular appearance. The increased prominence of the body landmarks can be noted at the ribs, xiphoid process, iliac crest, tips of the vertebrae, and the wings of the scapula.

Fat is redistributed from the periphery to the center of the body. Loss of fat is evident, especially on the dorsal aspects of the hands and on the arms, calves, legs, and buttocks. In contrast, there is an increase in truncal fat, especially on the abdomen.

## Skin

The skin undergoes a generalized loss of water; there is drying and scaling called xerosis, which is often accompanied by pruritus and flaking. Several factors account for these characteristic age changes. Long-term environmental exposure produces a so-called tanning effect. The sweat (apocrine) and sebaceous glands atrophy, further decreasing the skin lubrication. Absence of perspiration in the axilla and groin is a common finding and does not necessarily connote dehydration in older people. Hormonal changes, specifically diminished production of thyroxin, estrogens, and androgens, contribute to drying and thinning of the skin. Some of these changes can be prevented or reversed by the use of systemic estrogens.

The xerosis, coupled with diminished elasticity and loss of subcutaneous tissue, accounts for the skin changes seen on the face of older adults. Creases and wrinkle lines appear, especially in lines of habitual expression and motor use. The frown lines on the forehead become more prominent. Crow's feet appear as fanwise wrinkles emanating from

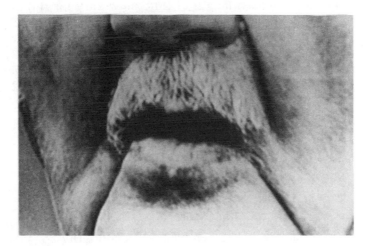

**FIGURE 5.2 Crease and wrinkle lines commonly seen around the nose and mouth.**

With permission from videotape "Physical Assessment of the Aged Person" produced by Herbert H. Lehman College, Department of Nursing, in association with Blue Hill Educational Systems, Inc., under sponsorship of Research Foundation of the City University of New York, 1975.

the lateral canthus of the eyes. Comma-shaped lines are seen on either side of the nose.

The facial skin becomes increasingly lax and subject to the effects of gravitational pull. Ptosis, or drooping of the eyelids, may be evident. The appearance of jowls on either side of the face and a double chin are further evidence of skin laxness.

Inspection may reveal characteristic changes in skin pigmentation in elderly whites. There is a decrease in the number and an uneven distribution of melanocytes. Keratin production decreases, and the small blood vessels become increasingly friable. These changes cause the skin on the face and neck to become more uniform in color and take on a white, opaque, putty-colored appearance (Balin, 1990). Areas of spotty pigmentation are commonly seen. Because of these age changes, assessment of skin color is not helpful in determining presence of anemia in the older person.

Atrophy and thinning of the skin on the back of the hands and forearms are also common. The subcutaneous veins may appear more prominent, and there may be evidence of increased bruising and telangiectasias.

The decrease in total body water and connective tissue changes result in diminished skin turgor. Skin turgor is best determined by gently pinching the skin over a bony prominence. Decreased turgor is evidenced in the increased length of time necessary for the pinched skin fold to return to the resting position. Assessment of turgor is not helpful in determining hydration in an older adult, because turgor may appear to be decreased in an adequately hydrated older client.

There are several skin lesions commonly seen in older people (see Figures 5.3 and 5.4). They are listed and described in Table 5.2.

## Hair

There is a generalized loss of hair from the periphery to the center of the body. The hair on the extremities as well as axillary and pubic hair diminishes. Loss of scalp hair (balding) is genetically determined and occurs from the center to the periphery of the scalp. It is not uncommon to see loss of the outer third of the eyebrows in older men.

The hair may thin out and become less wavy or kinky. The appearance of chin whiskers in women occurs secondarily to hormonal

---

**FIGURE 5.3 (A) Lentigines (liver spots) seen on the back of the hand. (B) Acrochordons (cutaneous tags). (C) Ichthyosis seen in the arm.**

Courtesy of Dermatology Division, Albert Einstein College of Medicine, New York.

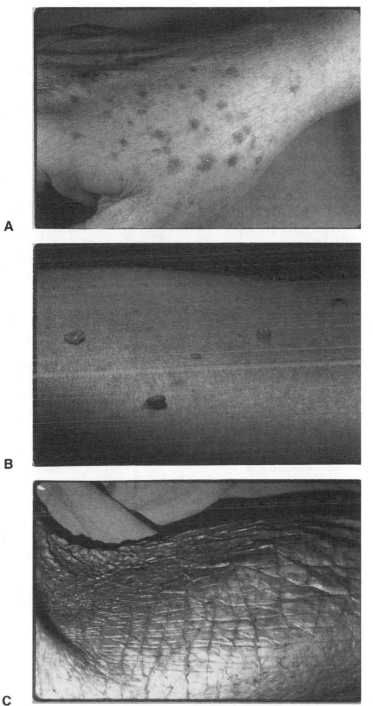

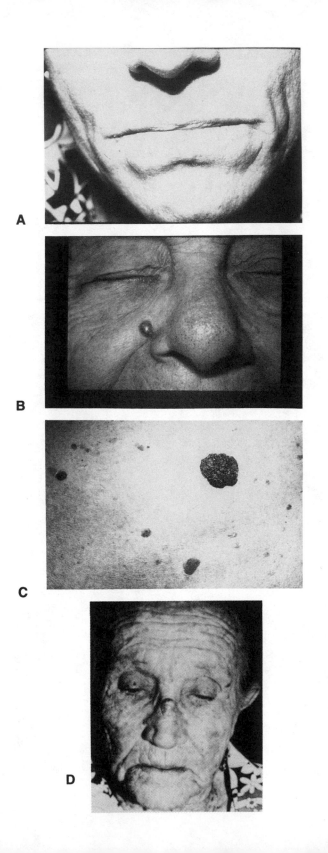

A

B

C

D

**TABLE 5.2 Skin Lesions Common in Older People**

| Skin Lesions | Description |
|---|---|
| Lentigines (liver spots) | Discrete or confluent freckles that increase in numbers with age. They are seen on the face, arms, hands, and legs. |
| Ichthyosis | Fish scale appearance of the skin, resulting from hypertrophy of the horny layers of the epidermis. |
| Acrochordons (skin tags) | Soft, flesh-colored, pedunculated lesions seen on the neck and in the axilla. |
| Actinic or senile keratosis, or warts | Papular, oval, brown or black lesions evident on the side of the nose and along crease lines of the head, neck, and trunk. These lesions are precancerous and require treatment. |
| Seborrheic keratosis | Some may appear as dome-shaped, black, and shiny, while others appear raised, yellowish, and greasy. Most commonly seen at the hair line, and on the neck, chest, and back. Also precancerous leisons. |
| Venous lakes | Bluish-black papular, vascular lesions, single or or multiple, seen on the exposed areas of the face, neck, and ears. |
| Senile ectasias (senile or cherry angiomas) | Red-purple lesions, 1 to 5 mm in size, seen on the upper chest and trunk. |
| Basal cell carcinoma (epithelioma) | A common malignant lesion in aged adults. Raised, red "T-zone" of the face—the forehead, eyelids, cheeks, nose, and lips. It most often feels hard on palpation. |

changes. Although graying is the most commonly seen hair color change, some people experience a lightening in color, or the hair may take on a yellow-green appearance. On palpation, the hair may feel coarse and dry. Senile xerosis of the scalp is a common finding in older people.

## Feet

The increased incidence of foot and vascular problems in older people dictates the need for a careful physical examination of the lower extremities. The skin should be warm and of normal texture. The color should be even and congruent with the general skin tones.

**FIGURE 5.4 (A) Venous lake seen on the lower lip. (B) Basal cell carcinoma (epithelioma) on the left side of the nose. (C) Seborrheic keratosis on the left cheek. (D) Multiple actinic or senile keratosis on the nose and face.**

Courtesy of Dermatology Division, Albert Einstein College of Medicine, New York.

Examination of the feet includes inspection of the skin and nails. Corns, painful circular areas of thickened skin in areas of the foot where skin is normally thin, and calluses, thickened skin usually on the sole of the foot, may be seen, especially in areas of bony configuration. Fungus infections often appear as fissures between the toes. Accentuation of previous foot deformities is a common occurrence and is manifested in such deformities as hallux valgus with a bunion, hammer toe, and splay foot. The nails become increasingly brittle and thickened, with peeling often occurring (see Figure 5.5). Fungal infections of the nails are a common finding. These changes cause distortions in the shape of the nails, such as Ram's Horn deformities, and increase the incidence of ingrown toenails (see Figure 5.6).

## Implications for Practice

As in all areas, the thoroughness of the assessment serves as the basis on which to judge whether specific findings are normal for the older client's age or if they represent deviations from the norm. Only within the context of a full data base can the assessment provide a sound rationale for an appropriate plan.

It is important to assess what age-related changes in general appearance and skin mean to the older client's self-concept. Changes that may

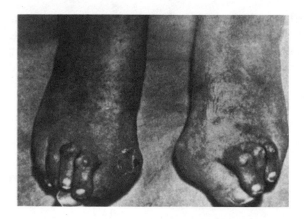

**FIGURE 5.5. Bilateral hallus valgus with bunions and multiple corns.**

From Silberstein, J.S. (1977). Extremities. In Prior, J.A., & Silberstein, J.S. (Eds.). *Physical Diagnosis*, 5th Ed. St. Louis: C.V. Mosby Co. Reprinted with permission.

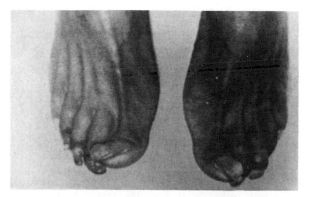

**FIGURE 5.6. Fungal infections of the toenails (onychomycosis).**

From Silberstein, J.S. (1977). Extremities. In Prior, J.A., & Silberstein, J.S. (Eds.) *Physical Diagnosis*, 5th Ed. St. Louis: C.V. Mosby Co. Reprinted with permission.

seem minor to the practitioner may be of crucial importance to the older person within the context of the individual's lifestyle and values. Clients' reactions to perceived changes in body image have implications for every aspect of their lives. Older people need to be given an opportunity to express anger and shock with the physical changes they are experiencing.

During each interaction, maintenance of a positive self-image should be supported. Optimal personal appearance should be encouraged to the extent that this is important to the client. People may limit what they do if they have negative feelings about how they look. Intervention, in these instances, should be directed toward assisting the older client to feel more positive about him or herself and preventing unnecessary social isolation.

In relation to skin care, the older client should be counseled regarding the need to dress in warm clothing and to avoid discomfort and chilling in a cold environment. Skin dryness is often associated with pruritus, excoriation, and cracking. Frequent application of effective and economical lubricants and emollients should be recommended because they act to hold water in the cells. The use of mild soaps or soap substitutes, such as Alpha-Keri bath oil, can be encouraged. Use of strong soaps that remove natural oils from the skin should be avoided. Appropriate skin care includes patting the skin almost dry after bathing, followed by immediate application of a cream. Sun screens can retard age changes when used at an early age. Their effectiveness in older people has, however, not been tested. If the older client requires a period of bedrest, however short, immediate preventive measures should be instituted, including the use of assessment instruments to ascertain risk for developing pressure ulcers (Braden & Bergstrom, 1989).

Foot care is an important area for counseling and intervention in the elderly client because of the common occurrence of bone, joint, and peripheral vascular changes. The nurse should ascertain whether the client and/or a family member are knowledgeable about foot care. It is especially important for older people to inspect their feet several times a week and that the toenails be cut correctly. Skin and nail problems may be of sufficient severity to require special care, in which case a referral to a podiatrist is appropriate. The wearing of well-fitting, supportive, leather shoes should be recommended, and the client should be told that walking is the best form of exercise for the feet.

## REFERENCES

Balin, A. (1990). Aging of human skin. In Hazzard, W., Andres, R., Bierman, E., & Blass, J. (Eds.) *Principles of Geriatric Medicine and Gerontology*. New York: McGraw-Hill Information Services Company.

Braden B., & Bergstrom, N. (1989). Clinical utility of the Braden Scale for predicting pressure sore risk. *Decubitus*, 18: 44–46, 50–51.

Fulmer, T. (1989). Mistreatment of elders: Assessment, diagnosis and intervention. *Nursing Clinics of North America, 24*, 707–716.

Kuhn, M. M. (1991). *Pharmaco-therapeutics: a Nursing Process Approach*. Philadelphia: F.A. Davis Company.

Schank, M. J. (1977). A survey of the well elderly: Their foot problems, practices, and needs. *Journal of Gerontological Nursing, 3*(6), 10.

## SUGGESTED READINGS

Braden, B., & Bryant, R. (1990). Innovations to prevent and treat pressure ulcers. *Geriatric Nursing, 10*, 182–186.

Chenitz, C., Stone, J., & Salisbury, S. (1991). *Clinical gerontological nursing: A guide to advanced practice*. Philadelphia: W.B. Saunders Co.

Finch, C., & Schneider, E. (Eds.). (1985). *Handbook of the biology of aging*. New York: Van Nostrand Reinhold.

Gilchrest, B. A. (1986). Skin disease in the elderly. In Calkins, E., Davis, D., & Ford, A. (Eds.), *The practice of geriatrics*. Philadelphia: W.B. Saunders Co.

Grove, G. (1989). Physiologic changes in older skin. *Clinical Geriatric Medicine, 5*, 115–120.

Jones, P., & Millman, A. (1990). Wound healing and the aged patient. *Nursing Clinics of North America, 25,* 263–277.

Kligman, A., & Graham, J. (1989). The psychology of appearance in the elderly. *Clinical Geriatric Medicine, 5,* 213–217.

Leaf, A. (1984). Dehydration in the elderly. *New England Journal of Medicine, 311,* 791–782.

Sauer, G. (1988). *Geriatric dermatology. Manual of skin diseases* (Ed. 6). Philadelphia: J.B. Lippincott.

# 6

# Assessment of Changes in the Eye, Ear, Nose, Mouth, and Neck

## HISTORY

The sensory organs constitute the body's primary mechanisms for experiencing and communicating with the environment. Sensory changes are a major source of morbidity in old age. Older people are often aware of and report even small changes in the sensory modalities of vision, hearing, smell, taste, and food intake. On the other hand, older people who expect some sensory changes as a normal aspect of aging may minimize symptoms or see symptoms as being of no interest to the practitioner or of no consequence to their health history. The nurse, therefore, needs to question the client carefully in order to gain as complete a data base as possible.

### Client Profile

The client profile, which includes data on living environment, activity, nutrition, etc., provides a rich source of data indicative of changes in the functioning of the eyes, ears, nose, throat, mouth, and neck. The client's present and past occupation may suggest contact with environmental irritants that affect sensory function. For example, a work environment with a high level of noise pollution places the older person at greater risk of developing a neuronal hearing deficit. At home, the client may demonstrate the presence of a hearing deficit by raising the volume of the television.

Clients should be questioned as to reasons for changes in activity patterns. For example, limiting the distance they are willing to drive a car or eliminating night driving are often attributable to decreased visual acuity and glare tolerance. Altered patterns of interaction with peers, such as decreasing attendance at senior citizen club functions, may be attributable to worsening hearing or vision.

Even when the level of social interaction is sustained, questions should be asked to determine whether sensory deficits diminish the level of satisfaction derived from these interactions. Changes in an older person's perception of his or her health and age may also reflect onset of sensory deficits. Self-perception can easily be determined by asking such questions as: "How would you describe your health?" and "Do you feel young, middle-aged, or old?" Findings suggest that older people who experience sensory deficits in hearing and vision are more likely to feel in poorer health and to feel older (Shanas, Townsend, Wedderburn et al., 1968).

Obtaining a detailed description of a 24-hour nutritional intake is an essential aspect of the health history (see Chapter 8 for a more complete discussion of nutritional assessment). Changes in appetite and food preferences may be attributable to a wide variety of causes, the most common of which are deficits in taste and smell, poor dentition or ill-fitting dentures, and altered ability to chew and swallow food. Changes in the milieu in which meals are eaten may also be related to sensory changes. The older person whose hearing has declined may be less willing to sit and converse at the family dinner table.

A history of the nutritional components of the older person's diet may reveal vitamin and mineral deficits or excesses that can be the cause of, or contribute to, pathology. For example, both vitamin A deficiency and vitamin D excess result in visual disturbances. Vitamin A deficiency is more common in people who have deficient protein intake and use extensive laxatives (Bartoshuk, Refkin, Markes et al., 1986, pp. 51–57).

## Past Health History

The health maintenance history should include frequency, results, and last date of vision and hearing testing and dental care. For people who wear glasses or a hearing aid, the provider should determine when the most recent prescription was obtained and any problems with the client's ability to manipulate an aid, for example to change the batteries. A history of repeated childhood episodes of otitis media may help to explain hearing deficits in the older client. Important also is a detailed information of past and current medications that may cause iatrogenic sensory deficits. Table 6.1 lists medications commonly used to treat chronic diseases of older people and shows how these medications can adversely affect sensory function.

A history of past illnesses should detail type of illness, past treatment, and any residual sensory deficits. Obviously, a past or current history of such chronic diseases as diabetes, hypertension, arteriosclerosis, or cerebral vascular accident suggests the possibility that the client may demonstrate concomitant visual or auditory signs and symptoms. Arteriosclerosis, for example, may result in hearing deficit. Family history may reveal incidence of familial tendency toward such eye diseases as cataracts, glaucoma, or senile macular degeneration.

# REVIEW OF SYSTEMS

## Eye

Many people report visual changes thought to occur as a result of the aging process. Older people require more light to see clearly and report requiring a longer time to adapt to light changes. They may complain of requiring an increased light intensity for reading, or they may report initiating the use of a night light to facilitate entering a darkened room. The client may complain of a decreased ability to drive at night because of a decreased tolerance to the direct lighting of oncoming traffic.

Several physiologic changes account for these deficits. With increasing age, there is an increase in the absolute light threshold. Older people require two to three times more light to see than younger adults and the transmission of light through the lens drops over 65% between the ages of 25 and 60 (Stoehr & Knapp, 1989). Dark adaptation diminishes and it can take the elderly person over 30 minutes to achieve full dark adaption. As the lens yellows with increasing age, color discrimination becomes less acute, especially in the blue, green, and violet color tones. The pupils decrease in size and ability to constrict (senile miosis), further limiting the amount of light reaching the retina. These deficits may not be corrected by increased lighting because of a decreased tolerance to glare secondary to increased lens opacity. The problem is improved only by an increase in indirect lighting.

It is not uncommon for older clients to report difficulty in perceiving objects at the periphery of their range of vision. For example, with peripheral field deficits, clients may report such changes as bumping

**TABLE 6.1. Adverse Effects on Sensory Function of Medications Commonly Used to Treat Chronic Diseases of Older People**

| Health Problem Medication | | Side Effects | | | |
|---|---|---|---|---|---|
| Generic name | Trade name | Eye | Ear | Nose | Mouth |
| **Anxiety** | | | | | |
| Chlordiazepoxide | Librium | Blurred vision | | | |
| Diazepam | Valium | Blurred vision | | | |
| Alprazolam | Xanex | | Lightheadedness | | Dry mouth |
| **Arthritis** | | | | | |
| Salicylates | Aspirin | Visual disturbances | Tinnitus | | |
| Ibuprofen | Motrin | Visual disturbances | | | |
| Indomethecin | Indocin | Corneal deposits; retinal disturbances | | | |
| Corticosteroids | | Cataracts; glaucoma | | | |
| **Heart disease** | | | | | |
| Digitalis | Digoxin | Visual disturbances | Tinnitus | | Dry mouth |
| Thiazides | Diuril | | Tinnitus; Decreased hearing | | Dry mouth |
| Furosemide | Lasix | | | | |
| **Glaucoma** | | | | | |
| Cholinergics | Timoptic | Miosis; diminished light adaptation; increased tearing | | Rhinorrhea | Increased salivation |
| **Hypertension** | | | | | |
| Captopril | Capoten | | | | Loss of taste |
| Nifedipine | Procardia | | | Nasal congestion Epistaxis | Dry mouth |
| Methyldopa | Aldomet | | | | |
| **Infections** | | | | | |
| Streptomycin | | | Tinnitus; Decreased hearing; Meniere's syndrome | | |
| Neomycin | | | | | |
| Kanamycin | | | | | |
| Gentamycin | | | Vertigo | | |
| Furandantin | Macrodantin | | | | Anorexia |
| Muscle cramps | | | | | |
| Quinine | Quinamm | Visual disturbances | Tinnitus; Vertigo | | |

into objects, unsteady gait, or having a diminished visual field when driving. While peripheral field deficits may be due to common physiologic changes, the practitioner always should consider the possibility of increased ocular pressure. Central field deficits are not normal sequelae of aging and may occur from senile macular degeneration, which produces central vision loss (scotoma) without peripheral field impairments. Retinal tears or detachments can also cause partial scotoma's (Stoehr & Knapp, 1989).

The most common alteration in vision is presbyopia, or farsightedness (Stefansson, 1990). People experiencing presbyopia report difficulty focusing on nearby objects and need to hold objects or reading matter at "arm's length." They may also report inadequacies in previously prescribed corrective lenses. Presbyopia is caused by degenerative changes in the crystalline lens. The lens becomes less transparent, the hydration of the lens decreases, and it loses elasticity, thereby diminishing its accommodative property.

Complaints of irritation, burning, or the sensation of a foreign body in the eye result from dryness of the eyes and decreased tear secretions (Stefansson, 1990). On the other hand, the older client may complain of increased tearing. Though the amount of lacrimation is thought to decrease with age, overflow of tears may be due to an impaired drainage of the ductal system. The conjunctiva becomes thinner and increasingly fragile with age. The client may require the instillation of artificial tears in the form of eye drops to keep the cornea adequately moistened. If the older person is exposed to environmental irritants such as cold, wind, dust, or air pollution, the occurrence of increased tearing and an uncomfortable sensation of sand or grit in the eye may suggest the presence of an inflammation in the conjunctiva requiring further evaluation. A history of diplopia, inflammation, pain, or photo-phobia should not occur as part of the normal aging process (Applegate, Miller, Elam et al., 1987).

Cataracts and glaucoma are the most common diseases affecting vision in older people. A cataract is an opacity of the crystalline lens. The symptoms depend on the location, size, and stage of development of the lesion. In early stages of the development of the cataract, the client may report an improvement in near vision because increased lens density temporarily improves refraction. The most commonly reported alterations, however, are progressive unilateral or bilateral painless loss of vision. Older people may delay reporting symptoms under the erroneous belief that cataracts need to "ripen" before surgery can be considered. Actually, the decision as to when to surgically remove a cataract depends primarily on the degree to which the cataract interferes with performance of desired activities. Cataract surgery is associated with improvements in both vision and functional status (Stefansson, 1990; Applegate et al., 1987).

Glaucoma, a disease of the eye caused by an increase in intraocular pressure, is the second most common cause of legal blindness among people over 65. In the early stages of chronic, open angle glaucoma, the most common form, no symptoms are evident and diagnosis is made by use of repeated visual field testing, fundoscopic examination, and measurement of intra-ocular pressure. Because measurement of intra-ocular pressure using tonometry examination often yields false negative readings, tonometry alone is not a useful tool for either detecting or following the progression of glaucoma (Applegate et al., 1987). As at any age, acute, narrow angle glaucoma is a medical emergency presenting with symptoms of pain in and around the eye, perception of halos around lights, clouding of vision, and impairment of peripheral vision often associated with naseau and vomiting.

Senile macular degeneration is a disease of the eye which presents with a gradual, painless loss of central vision and loss of detailed vision needed to read (Stoehr & Knapp, 1989; Mezey & Grisso, 1989). Peripheral vision is rarely affected and the degeneration rarely causes total blindness. If macular degeneration is suspected, the patient is often asked to assess change of vision at home using a grid with a central dot (Figure 6.1). Progression of symptoms is monitored by determining the degree to which the lines on the grid appear wavy or blurred.

Visual changes may also accompany acute episodes of illness. Transient blindness or unilateral reduction in visual fields can accompany a transient ischemic attack (TIA) (Stoehr & Knapp, 1989). Fluctuation in vision often occurs as a result of increased blood glucose in the diabetic.

## Ear

The most common hearing deficit in older age is presbycusis, a sensory-neural hearing loss that progresses from a high tone loss to a generalized loss of hearing in all frequencies. It has been estimated that close to one in three people 75 and over experience hearing losses in the most important frequencies (Moseicki et al., 1985). Most speech takes place in the range of 500 to 2,000 Hz. Sounds such as s, th, j, k, and f are heard in higher frequencies (Rees & Duckert, 1990). Because older people lose the ability to perceive pitch above 4,000 Hz, they have difficulty in hearing these sounds. This increase in sound threshold also causes difficulty in understanding words spoken in the normal speaking range. There is often a concomitant decrease in speech discrimi-

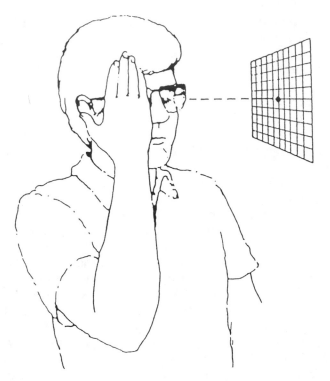

**FIGURE 6.1 Grid that can be used at home to assess progression of senile macular degeneration. Patient examines Amsler's grid with each eye. Grid is placed on wall at comfortable distance normally used for reading. If patient requires reading glasses or bifocals, these are worn.**

From Editorial. Laser Treatment for Eye Disease. *Journal of the American Medical Association*, 1983; *250*(18), p. 2508. Copyright 1983, American Medical Association. Reprinted with permission.

nation that is evident, especially when the client tries to carry on a conversation in a noisy environment, when speech is rapid, or when the client needs to discriminate between phonetically similar words, for example words that begin with f, g, s, t and z. Environmental sounds may also be incorrectly identified.

Because presbycusis presents as a gradual hearing deficit, the older person has often learned to partially compensate by facing people directly in a conversation, lip reading, and restricting conversations to those between him or herself and one other person. Lastly, the practitioner should be aware that tinnitus, vertigo, ear pain, and evidence of inflammation are not sequelae of normal aging.

## Nose

While age changes manifested in the nose are not of major importance, older people report a decreased ability to identify and discriminate between odors. This is due to a progressive decrease in the sense of smell (anosmia). Complaints of dryness of the skin around the nares are frequent. The commonly reported symptoms of rhinorrhea, sneezing, and post nasal discharge suggest the presence of vasomotor rhinitis secondary to atrophic changes in the mucous membrane and increasing susceptibility to nasal irritation. These symptoms may be accompanied by epistaxis, especially following periods of sneezing and nose blowing. Epistaxis may also result from hypertension or other arterial vessel changes.

## Mouth

Changes in the teeth, tongue, musculature of the mouth, and sense of taste will be reflected in alterations in eating habits, appetite, and nutritional intake. Approximately 40% of people over the age of 65 are edentulous (Miller et al., 1987). Changes in the type of food eaten may suggest difficulty with dentition or alterations in sense of taste. While taste sensation diminishes with age, with the decrease in ability to taste sweets being especially pronounced, more recent studies suggest that such changes are more modest in the well elderly and are compounded by disease, medications, and poor oral hygiene (Spitzer, 1988; Bartoshuk et al., 1986, pp. 51–55). Older people may consume increasing amounts of sugar to compensate for this deficit.

The complaint of dry mouth, known as xerostosis, and a bad taste in the mouth are common. While these symptoms usually result from iatrogenic causes such as medications (Baum & Ship, 1990), they may also be caused by atrophic changes in the mucous membranes and salivary glands, or they may be symptoms of gingival disease. A complete dental history, including date of last dental visit, should be elicited. If a client wears partial or complete dentures, a detailed history as to the length of time worn, comfort, type of food eaten, and satisfaction with the fit of the prosthesis should be ascertained. Older clients may complain of pain on movement of the jaw due to temporomandibular joint degeneration. Bleeding gums and hoarseness are not seen as normal sequelae of aging.

## Neck

The review of systems in relation to the neck should be unchanged in older adults. Symptoms of sore throat, hoarseness, dysphagia, or stiff neck do not occur as normal age changes.

# PHYSICAL EXAMINATION

## Eye

The examination of the eyes of older people begins, as with any age group, with a determination of visual acuity. Each eye should be assessed separately, under normal room illumination, and with the other eye completely covered. The practitioner should note whether the examination is with or without spectacle correction (Stoehr & Knapp, 1989). The Snellen chart tests visual acuity at 20 feet. Newspaper or other reading material, or a standardized method, such as a Jaeger Card, should be used to determine near vision. This is especially important since older people are more likely to have presbyopia.

For an accurate determination of visual acuity, the light source should originate from behind the client. The client should not be rushed, because speed is not a factor in assessing acuity. In the absence of any opacity of the clear structures of the eye, visual acuity is an indicator of the function of the second cranial nerve. (See Chapter 12, Table 12.1 for differences in cranial nerve assessment techniques and findings in the older client.) The confrontation test will provide a gross estimate of visual field and is helpful in confirming field defects. Normal visual fields are also indicative of intact second cranial nerve function.

Inspection of the eye often reveals some common age changes. The skin around the orbit of the eye may be darkened. Enopthalmus, the recession of the eyeball into the orbit, may be evident due to decreased orbital fat. Tearing is often evident. Carefully observe the lid for drainage, crusting, or irritation. Basal cell carcinomas have a high rate of occurence in the inner third of the lower lid (Stoehr & Knapp, 1989). Muscle flaccidity or atrophy of the eyelids can result in a senile entropian, an inturning, or ectropian, an eversion, of the lower lid (see Figure 6.2). Entropian may be accompanied by trichiasis, a condition where the eyelashes turn in and brush the conjunctiva. If this condition causes inflammation, it will require surgical correction. The skin folds of the upper lids may appear more prominent, and pouches may be visible under the eye due to herniation of fat through the weakened muscle.

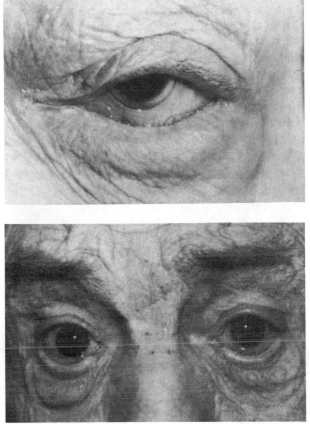

**FIGURE 6.2 (A) Senile entropian and trichiasis of the lower eyelid. (B) Senile ectropian of the lower eyelids. Note also the loss of the outer third of the eyebrow, the prominence of the skin folds of the upper lid, and the pouches under the eyes.**

Courtesy of H. Malpica, Department of Ophthalmology, Montefiore Hospital and Medical Center/Albert Einstein College of Medicine, New York.

The conjunctiva of the eye may appear paler than in younger adults. The presence of fat deposition will result in several commonly seen age changes. The conjunctiva and sclera may take on a yellow appearance. Xanthelasmas, cutaneous deposition of lipids, are seen in the inner portion of the eye or on the upper or lower lids and clear to yellowish fleshy looking areas (pingueculae) may be seen on the conjunctive, either nasal or temporal to the cornea (Stoehr & Knapp, 1989). An arcus senilis, an opaque chalky white or greenish-yellow arc or ring, is seen partially or totally encircling the periphery of the cornea. None of these fatty deposits affect vision (see Figure 6.3).

The iris may appear pale and have a stippled brown appearance due to pigment degeneration. The pupils can appear smaller in size, unequal, and irregular in shape. Reaction to light and accommodation, reflecting third cranial nerve function, should be present and symmetrically equal but may be less brisk. The pupil will have a keyhole shape

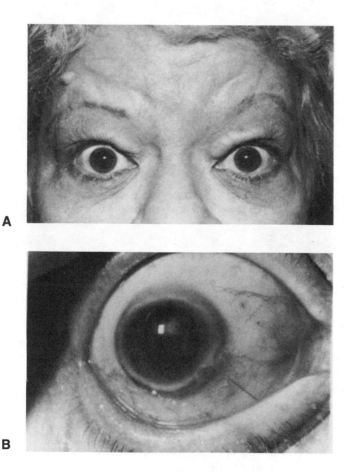

**FIGURE 6.3 (A) Bilateral xanthelasmas of the upper lids. (B) Arcus senilis totally encircling the cornea.**

Courtesy of H. Malpica, Department of Ophthalmology, Montefiore Hospital and Medical Center/Albert Einstein College of Medicine, New York.

following an iridectomy in people who have undergone surgery for removal of cataracts or treatment of glaucoma (see Figure 6.4)

There should be no alteration in the shape or clarity of the cornea. Any abnormality of the cornea requires referral for further evaluation. A pterygium, a clear or yellowish area seen in the cornea adjacent to the limbus may cause visual deficits. When testing the corneal reflex (fifth cranial nerve), a prolonged stimulation may be necessary to elicit a response. Once elicited, however, the response should be brisk and consensual.

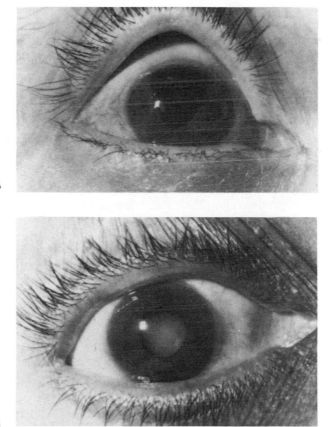

**FIGURE 6.4 (A) Partial iridectomy. (B) Cataract.**

Courtesy of H. Malpica, Department of Ophthalmology, Montefiore Hospital and Medical Center/Albert Einstein College of Medicine, New York.

Prior to beginning the fundoscopic examination, it is desirable to dilate the pupil. This is especially necessary in older clients who evidence increased pupillary constriction and decreased tolerance to glare. Dilating the pupil is, however, contraindicated in clients who have a history or symptoms suggestive of glaucoma, since dilation may precipitate an episode of acute glaucoma. If dilation of the pupil with medication is contraindicated, just darkening the examination room may be sufficient.

On beginning the fundoscopic examination, the practitioner should be aware that some degree of cataract development is expected in almost all people over 70. A cataract may partially or totally obstruct the red reflex and visualization of the fundus. The number 10 lens of the opthalmoscope can help to highlight the opacity against the red reflex (Mezey & Grisso, 1989). The appearance will depend on the stage of development and its location in the lens. Centrally placed cataracts may appear as milky white opacities when viewed through the pupil. The degree to which the cataract obscures the macular provides some indication of the cataract's density (Mezey & Grisso, 1989). Other types of cataracts will appear as areas of diffuse pigmentation or as spider webs and will give off a black reflection.

The fundus may reveal certain characteristic age changes. The retina and optic disc normally appear paler than in younger adults. The arteries and veins often do not show their customary 2 to 3 ratio. A silver wire and tortuous appearance to the arteries is evidence of an atherosclerotic process. Papilledema is rarely evident in people over 70, and therefore absence of this sign does not rule out pathology. On fundoscopic examination the practitioner may note signs of macular degeneration such as alteration in pigmentation and configuration in and near the macular. Small, discrete yellowish "freckles" near the macular (macular drusen) may be noted. Macular drusen that coalesce may be early evidence of macular degeneration (Stoehr & Knapp, 1989).

The practitioner will need to be familiar with the fundoscopic manifestations of three systemic chronic diseases: hypertension, arteriosclerosis, and diabetes. While it is not expected that every practitioner will be proficient in diagnosis of fundoscopic findings, ability to recognize abnormalities will enhance early detection and permit more objective follow-up of clients with pre-existing pathology.

Retinal hypertension presents as a narrowing and constricting of the vessels with the presence of hemorrhages and exudates. The findings are recorded as grades ranging from 1 to 4 as follows:

Grade 1    Narrowing of the terminal branches of the vessels.
Grade 2    General narrowing of the vessels with severe local constriction.

Grade 3   To the preceding signs are added striate hemorrhage and soft exudates.

Grade 4   Papilledema is added to the preceding signs, but may not be evident in people over 70 (Applegate et al., 1987).

Arteriosclerosis is usually characterized by signs of arteriolar-venular (A-V) nicking. The grading for retinal arteriolar sclerosis is as follows:

Grade 1   Thickening of the vessels with slight depression of veins at A-V crossings.

Grade 2   Definite A-V crossing changes; moderate local sclerosis.

Grade 3   Venule beneath the arteriole is invisible; severe local sclerosis and segmentation.

Grade 4   To the preceding signs are added venous obstruction and arteriolar obliteration (Mezey & Grisso, 1989).

Diabetes results in severe visual impairment. Microaneurysms around the macula and the appearance of white or waxy exudates are characteristic of diabetic retinopathy. Presence of cataracts or glaucoma is an indication for screening for diabetes mellitus.

Measurement of intraocular pressure (IOP) can be accomplished through tonometry examination or referral to an opthamologist. Normal IOP averages about 16.1 mm Hg. and an increase in IOP is suggestive of glaucoma (Mezey & Grisso, 1989). While a positive tonometry examination is indicative of increased intraocular pressure, a normal tonometry reading cannot be construed as indicating that pressure is not elevated.

## Ear

Inspection of the ears may demonstrate commonly seen aged skin changes. Sagging and continued deposition of cartilage over the life cycle cause the earlobe to elongate and alter the shape of the auditory canal. The skin of the ear may appear dry and scratch marks will suggest the presence of senile pruritus. Otoscopic examination includes visualization of the auditory canal, tympanic membrane, ossicles, and light reflex. An increase in cerumen accumulation is a common cause of acute hearing loss in older adults and may also obscure landmarks in the middle ear. When visualized, landmarks may appear unchanged from those seen in younger adults. A thickening of the tympanic membrane and a slight diminution in the intensity of the light reflex constitute a normal age variation.

Testing of hearing reflects adequacy of eighth cranial nerve function. The use of the Weber and Rinne tests provides a gross assessment of

hearing. If prebycusis is present unilaterally, the Weber test will later-
alize to the unaffected ear and the Rinne test will show a normal ratio
of air to bone conduction with a generalized decrease in total hearing.
While older people initially experience deficits in hearing and differentiating high-pitched sounds, with increased age there is often a generalized loss of hearing in all frequencies.

Audiometry examinations should be a standard aspect of examination for all clients reporting hearing deficits. The hearing of older people
with presbycusis can be greatly enhanced by appropriate diagnosis and
treatment with a hearing aid.

## Nose

Because the nasal cartilage continues to grow, the nose may become
elongated and have a hooked appearance. Nasal speculum examination
may reveal an increase in nasal hair. If vasomotor rhinitis is present,
the mucous membrane of the nose will appear pale and the turbinates
may be boggy. Testing of the first cranial nerve function, the olfactory
nerve, often confirms a decrease in the sense of smell.

## Mouth

The physical examination of the mouth begins with inspection of
facial symmetry. Facial symmetry is a function of the seventh cranial
nerve and should not deteriorate with age. In the dentulous client,
examination begins with inspection of the lips and teeth. There may
be a generalized loss of the vermilion border of the lip. The number,
location, and condition of the teeth should be noted. The teeth may
show signs of staining, erosion, chipping, abrasions, and displacement
due to wearing of the superior surface and loss of dentine. If marked
erosion or attrition of the teeth has occurred, a malocclusion of the
teeth will be evident. The gums and mucous membranes of the mouth
appear increasingly thin and parchment-like. Atrophy of the sublingual
salivary glands and Stenson's ducts leading from the parotid glands
may be evident and is often accompanied by halitosis. The most common problem of the teeth is peri-dontal pathology. Atrophic gingivitis
presents as an enlargement of the interspaces between the teeth. If gingivitis progresses, the crown may become exposed, and the teeth appear longer. Hence, the increased toothiness seen in some older people.
Gingivitis also causes the teeth to become increasingly mobile and
diseased.

Atrophic changes are also evident on the tongue. Loss of the fungi-
form and filiform papillae on the lateral aspects of the tongue is espe-

cially common in older women. Varicosities of small blood vessels under the tongue, known as caviar spots, may also be evident (see Figure 6.5). Diminished taste sensation is attributable to atrophy of the taste buds and decreased sense of smell and indicates decreased function of the fifth and seventh cranial nerves. Full range of motion of the tongue should be present. The gag reflex may be slightly sluggish in comparison with younger adults.

Examination of the mouth of the edentulous older person should be done in two stages—with and without the dentures in place. With the dentures removed, the examiner will note a shrinkage of the lower face. Osteoporosis of the maxilla and mandible results in a diminishing of the distance between the nose and the chin. There is a "purse string" appearance to the upper and lower lips and an infolding of the mouth. A narrowing of the alveolar ridge may be evident, making the fitting of dentures increasingly difficult (see Figure 6.6).

The gums, mucous membrane, and hard and soft palate of the edentulous client should be carefully inspected and palpated. There

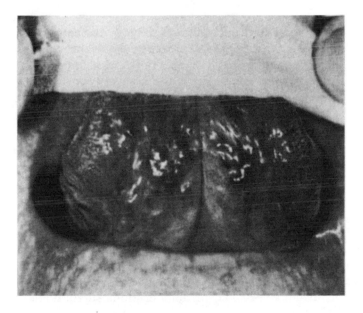

**FIGURE 6.5 Caviar spots seen under the tongue.**

From Colby, R.A., Kerr, D.A., & Robinson, H.D.G. [1971]. *Color Atlas of Oral Pathology.* Philadelphia: J.B. Lippincott Co.FIGURE 6.5 Caviar spots seen under the tongue. Reprinted with permission.

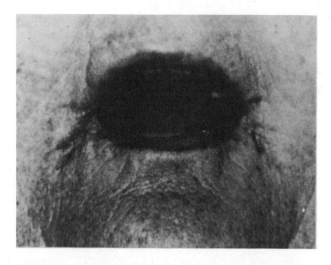

**FIGURE 6.6 Mouth changes commonly seen in the older people—purse-string appearance, loss of vermilion border, and Perleche.**

From Conrad, A.H. 1976. Dermatologic Disorders. In Steinberg, F.U. (Ed.) *Cowdry's The Care of the Geriatric Patient*, 5th Ed. St. Louis: C.V. Mosby Co. Reprinted with permission.

are certain lesions commonly seen in the mouths of denture wearers. Perleche refers to the downward folding and maceration at the corners of the mouth. This is often accompanied by cheilosis, which is characterized by macular papular lesions and fissures seen at the corners of the mouth. Upper dentures may create a suction chamber effect against the palate. This deformity results in the formation of papillary hyperplasia and is evidenced as warty lesions on the vault of the maxilla (see Figure 6.7).

The constant wearing of dentures can act as a source of friction and irritation in the mouth. "Denture sore mouth" is the term applied to a generalized inflammation of the denture-bearing area. Denture irritation or hyperplasia is a reactive inflammatory response characterized by a linear mass of scar tissue occurring between the denture flange and the edge of the adjacent bone. Decubiti, or dental sores, are localized lesions usually seen as central ulcerations surrounded by a raised and indurated border.

The edentulous client should next be examined with the dentures in place. Facial asymmetry, which may have been present with the dentures removed, should not be evident with the dentures in place. The

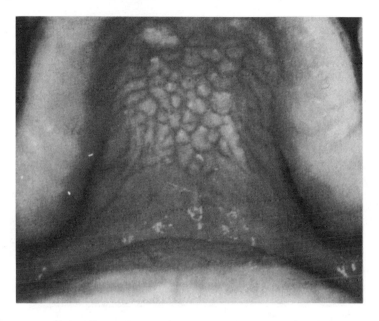

**FIGURE 6.7 Papillary hyperplasia on the vault of the maxilla.**
From Colby, R.A., Kerr, D.A., & Robinson, H.D.G. 1971. *Color Atlas of Oral Pathology.*
Philadelphia: J.B. Lippincott Co. Reprinted with permission.

fit of the denture plate should be firm and allow full range of motion of
the jaw. The jaw jerk reflex should be tested with the dentures in place,
since it may be difficult to elicit in the edentulous client.

The practitioner should observe the mouth for evidence of leukoplakia. Leukoplakia is a precancerous lesion seen in both dentulous
and edentulous older people. It will appear as white or whitish-gray
patches on the mucous membrane of the mouth and cheek, or on the
tongue and lips. The lesion often appears chalk white and has a "stuck
on" appearance (see Figure 6.8). Presence of leukoplakia requires
referral.

## Neck

On physical examination, inspection may reveal a shortening of the neck
due to osteoporosis of the cervical vertebrae. Two prominent wrinkle
lines are commonly seen at the lateral aspects of the neck. The thyroid is not normally palpable. The technique for palpation of the thy-

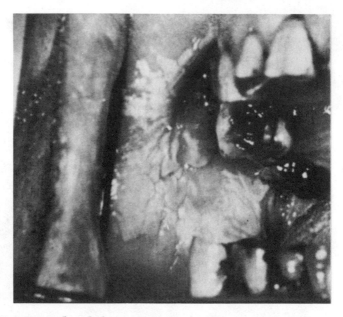

**FIGURE 6.8 Leukoplakia of the mouth.**

From Colby, R.A., Kerr, D.A., & Robinson, H.D.G. 1971. *Color Atlas of Oral Pathology.* Philadelphia: J.B. Lippincott Co. Reprinted with permission.

roid gland should be carried out lower in the neck in relation to the clavicle than is done in younger adults. Carefully assess for the presence of thyroid nodules and goiter.

Examination of the neck should include an assessment of the blood vessels in the region. Increased prominence of the right carotid artery pulsation may be evident due to a buckling of the innominate artery.

Auscultation of a carotid artery bruit warrants referral. Loss of subcutaneous tissue facilitates the determination of neck vein distension in older clients.

## IMPLICATIONS FOR PRACTICE

Sensory changes in vision, hearing, and taste affect multiple facets of the older person's daily life (Baum & Ship, 1990). For example, the condition of the mouth has implications for the client's verbal and nonverbal communication, appearance and self image, nutritional status, and respiratory function. Knowledge of normal age changes in these areas can be utilized to promote health, prevent accidents, and assist older people in appropriately modifying such activities of daily living as use of transportation, cooking, serving of meals, and managing household chores.

Ability to recognize normal age changes enables the practitioner to develop screening programs such as vision and hearing screening appropriate to specific population groups (U.S. Department of Health and Human Services, 1991). The comprehensive data base becomes the basis for prescribing health maintenance activities. The data base gathered at a time of good health serves as a base for comparison with data gathered at a later time and helps to differentiate between normal sequelae of aging and pathology.

The life satisfaction of older age correlates with feelings of good health and continued activity. Recognizing that older people are interested in their health and appearance, the practitioner can facilitate individual and group discussions of normal expected age changes that will enhance an understanding of the changes older people see occurring in themselves and in their peers.

# REFERENCES

Applegate, W., Miller, S., Elam, J. et al. (1987). Impact of cataract surgery with lens implantation on vision and physical function in elderly patients. *Journal of the American Geriatric Society, 257*(8), 164–166.

Bartoshuk, J., Refkin, B., Markes, L. et al. (1986). Taste and aging. *Journal of Gerontology, 41*, 51–57.

Baum, B., & Ship, J. (1990). The Oral Cavity. In Hazzard, W. et al. *Principles of geriatric medicine and gerontology*, Second Edition, (pp. 413–421). New York: McGraw Hill Publishing Co.

Mezey, M., & Grisso, J. A. (1989). Preventing dependence and injury: An approach to sensory changes. In Lavizzo-Mourey, R. Day, S., Diserens, D., & Grisso, J. A. *Practicing prevention for the elderly* (pp. 125–139). Philadelphia: Hanley & Belfus, Inc.

Miller et al. (1987). *The national survey of oral health in U.S. adults: 1985-1986.* DHHS (NIH) 87-2868. Washington, DC: U.S. Government Printing Office.

Moseicki, E. et al. (1985). Hearing loss in the elderly: An epidemiologic study of the Framingham heart study cohort. *Ear and Hearing, 6*, 184–187.

Rees, T., & Duckert, L. (1990). Auditory and vestibular dysfunction in aging. In Hazzard, W. et al. *Principles of geriatric medicine and gerontology*, Second Edition (pp. 432–444). New York: McGraw Hill Publishing Co.

Shanas, E., Townsend, P., Wedderburn, D. et al. (1968). The psychology of health. In Neugarten, B. L. (Ed.), *Middle age and aging* (p. 215). Chicago: University of Chicago Press.

Spitzer, M. (1988). Taste acuity in institutionalized and noninstitutionalized elderly men. *Journal of Gerontology, 43,* 71.

Stefansson, E. (1990). The eye. In Hazzard, W. et al. *Principles of geriatric medicine and gerontology,* Second Edition, (pp. 422–431). New York: McGraw Hill Publishing Co.

Stoehr, A., & Knapp, M. (1989). Physician checklist for visually impaired elderly in nursing homes. *Geriatrics, 44,* 87–91.

U.S. Department of Health and Human Services. (1991). *Healthy people 2000: National health promotion and disease prevention.* Rockville, MD: Public Health Service.

# SUGGESTED READINGS

Burke, M., & Walsh, M. (1992). *Gerontological nursing: Care of the frail elderly.* St. Louis: Mosby YearBook, Inc.

Chenitz, C., Stone, J., & Salisbury, S. (1991). *Clinical gerontological nursing: A guide to advanced practice.* Philadelphia: W. B. Saunders Company.

Corso, J. (1971) Sensory processes and age effects in normal adults. *Journal of Gerontology, 26,* 90–105.

Edsall, J., & Miller, L. (1978). Relationship between loss of auditory and visual acuity and social disengagement. *Nursing Research, 27*(5), 296–298.

Elipoulous, C. (1990). *Health assessment of the older adult* (2nd ed.). Redwood City, CA: Addison-Wesley Nursing.

Hazzard, W., Andres, R., Bierman, E., & Blass, J. (1990). *Principles of geriatric medicine and gerontology* (2nd ed.). New York: McGraw Hill Publishing Co.

Hearing impairment and elderly people: Background paper. (1986, May). Office of Technology Assessment. Congress of the United States. (OTA-BP-BA-30). Washington DC: U.S. Government Printing Office.

Kane, R., Ouslander, J., & Abrass, I. (1989). *Essentials of clinical geriatrics.* (2nd ed.). New York: McGraw-Hill Information Services Co., Health Professions Division.

Kahn, H., Leibowits, H., Ganley, J. et al. (1977). The Framingham eye study: Outline and major prevalence findings. *American Journal of Public Health, 106,* 17–32.

Orr, A. (Ed.). (1992). *Vision and Aging: Crossroads for Service Delivery.* NY: American Foundation for the Blind.

Rupp, R. R., Vaugh, G. R., & Lightfoot, R. K. (1986). Primary care for the hearing impaired: A changing picture. *Geriatrics, 41,* 74–84.

# 7

# Assessment of the Cardiac, Vascular, Respiratory, and Hematopoietic Systems

---

## HISTORY

### Client Profile

The client profile is a major source of information in assessment of the cardiac, vascular, respiratory, and hematopoietic systems. A general picture of exercise tolerance provides important clues as to the client's cardiac and respiratory reserve. Knowledge of typical activities such as how long it takes the client to make breakfast, dress, and shop provides information on current exercise tolerance. The client should be asked about changes in customary activities including how often he or she leaves the house in a week or about types of recreational activities. If activity changes have occurred, the individual should be questioned regarding the cause to determine if it is because of shortness of breath or exertional fatigue.

In order to accommodate respiratory or cardiovascular decline, clients may gradually alter their activities and thus not complain of exertional dyspnea, as they no longer physically overexert themselves. For example, such a person may spend most of the day sitting in a chair. To ascertain alterations in the client's prior exercise tolerance, the practitioner must ask questions about both recent and long-term change in activity. Recent changes usually indicate more acute problems. The client may describe activities that he or she would like to do but does not perform because of lack of stamina. Assessing the activity tolerance in the manner described previously will give the examiner a good data base from which to make judgments about cardiac reserve and other restraining factors such as arthritis or pulmonary disease. Some decrease in activity tolerance is an expected concomitant of the aging process. For example, the client may not be able to play three successive sets of tennis. It is not usual, however, for a person to become suddenly too tired to carry on the usual activities of daily living.

A description of the socialization of the individual is necessary, since a decrease in social activity may occur due to fatigue or dyspnea. The status of significant relationships and whether these are satisfying or stressful should be determined. Ascertaining whether the older client lives alone, is able to maintain usual relationships, and has the energy necessary to drive or walk to a friend's house will give important data on capacity for maintaining significant relationships and will tell the practitioner if there are people available to assist the client when help is needed.

The nutritional history is of prime importance for the assessment of the cardiac, vascular, respiratory, and hematopoietic systems. The client should carefully describe all the food consumed in a day as well as how the food is prepared. All condiments used should be enumerated, since people may not think of bouillon cubes or garlic salt as important aspects of the diet when, in fact, these foods add considerable sodium to the dietary intake.

The type and amount of fats ingested should be examined. Controversy exists concerning the effect of cholesterol intake on atherosclerotic disease progression in the elderly. When a low cholesterol diet is begun at a young age, the benefits are apparent. Elevated cholesterol levels develop slowly over many years, but recent evidence suggests lowering dietary intake of cholesterol in older people may alter the course of heart disease (Smith, Karmally, & Brown, 1987). The diet needs to be carefully examined to determine whether adequate amounts of iron are present to prevent development of iron deficiency anemia. Caloric requirements decrease with age, but the need for nutrients remains the same. Because many older individuals do not reduce calories appropriately, obesity is a common problem that places additional strain on the cardiovascular and respiratory systems. (See Chapter 8 on nutrition.)

It is important to know if there is a smoking history. Even if the client docs not currently smoke, the history includes data regarding all tobacco used in the past, such as cigarettes (filtered and unfiltered tobacco or marijuana), pipes, or cigars. Tobacco consumption is expressed in pack years, that is, number of packs smoked multiplied by the number of years smoked. Therefore, a person who smoked two packs of cigarettes for 40 years would have smoked 80 pack years ($2 \times 40 = 80$). Tobacco stains on the fingers can be a clue to current tobacco use.

A complete description of the home and community is essential in planning for the client with cardiovascular and respiratory deficits. Ascertaining whether the client has stairs to climb as well as determining the layout of the home and availability of facilities in the community are relevant to the profile. Chapter 13 further describes assessment of the home and community.

The history of family diseases and deaths related to the cardiovascular, respiratory, or hematopoietic systems is of interest to the practitioner. The practitioner should be cued to look for signs and symptoms of those illnesses for which there is a strong family history, for example, hyperlipidemia and hypertension.

## Past Health History

As with all clients, it is important to obtain the history of past cardiovascular, respiratory, and hematopoietic illnesses, hospitalizations, and surgeries. This history is likely to be quite long and complicated with the older client but, nevertheless, should be thoroughly obtained. Each area identified as a past health problem should be fully described.

Clients with longstanding cardiac or respiratory diseases will often take multiple medications. It is the rare client who carefully labels medications or who knows their exact names. If possible, ask the client to bring in all the medications being taken, both prescription and nonprescription. Always ask the client to show which pills are taken when, and for what reason the drug is prescribed. A question like, "Are you always able to take that medication every day?" may lead the client to describe when he or she skips the medication dosage. Commonly, older clients take medicines only when they feel ill or feel that they need the medicine. Only in a nonthreatening interview is the client likely to reveal the actual medication intake pattern.

# REVIEW OF SYSTEMS

## Cardiac System

Cardiac disease is the most common problem in the older person. It is therefore likely that the older client will now have, or has had in the past, some cardiac symptom. For each symptom, the examiner must determine the onset, duration, character, aggravating factors, relieving factors, associated findings, and current management.

High blood pressure is common in the older person. As many as 41% of the women and 33% of the men over 65 may be hypertensive (National Center for Health Statistics, 1987). The prevalence in elderly black men and women is even higher. The practitioner will therefore want to inquire about previous blood pressure readings or treatment. As with all age groups, hypertension is usually asymptomatic, but questions need to be asked regarding epistaxis or headaches.

A common complaint of the older client is light-headedness upon rising from a lying or sitting position. Orthostatic hypotension has been found in as many as 20% of outpatients. Postural hypotension may be caused by slowed baroreceptor reflex activity, medications, dehydration, or disease (Lipsitz, 1989). Post-prandial hypotension has also been reported.

When considering the possibility of a myocardial infarction (MI) in the older client, one must remember that the typical presence and pattern of chest pain may be absent. As many as 30% of older clients with an MI present without chest pain (Kannel, Dannenberg, & Abbott, 1985). In the older person with a "silent MI," the most common first and, at times, the only symptom is dyspnea. Gastrointestinal complaints such as nausea and vomiting and neurologic findings such as weakness, vertigo, confusion, or impaired consciousness may be other symptoms of a myocardial infarction.

Congestive heart failure (CHF) is a common sequela of heart disease and is frequently seen in older clients. To assess for the fluid retention of CHF it is particularly important to ask about weight gain and changes in fit of shoes, belts, or rings. If the client's vision is poor, he or she may not be able to see the scale and, therefore, the fit of clothes may be the primary indication of retention of fluid. Nocturia is a common complaint of the older person and the examiner must determine if the client first awakens and then thinks about going to the bathroom (not usually a symptom of CHF) or whether he or she wakes up due to a need to urinate (more often a symptom of CHF). The symptoms of dyspnea on exertion (DOE), paroxysmal nocturnal dyspnea (PND), orthopnea, previous history of CHF, and therapies for CHF should not be overlooked. The nurse must also remember that DOE and edema in the older person can be related to problems other than CHF, such as chronic obstructive pulmonary disease, restrictive lung disease, anemia, or cirrhosis.

## Vascular System

Vascular disease becomes more common with increasing age. The vascular history should include information about arterial and venous problems.

When considering arterial disease, it is important to determine the presence of symptoms caused by decreased perfusion of tissues supplied by a specific artery, for example, headaches with temporal artery disease and intermittent claudication or by paresthesia with femoral artery disease. If the occurrence of calf pain following exercise (intermittent claudication) is elicited, the practitioner should ascertain a detailed history of the amount of exercise that precipitates this symptom and any recent changes in the severity and frequency of occurrence. Older people frequently do not have the classical symptoms of pain, but rather present with related symptoms such as coldness, change in the color of skin, numbness, and/or paresthesias (Halperin, 1987). The individual may describe a loss of hair, shiny taut dry skin, and changes in the nails.

Venous disease of the lower extremities develops slowly and has a high incidence in the older population. Venous changes that the older client may report include varicosities, edema, inflammation, and ulcerations.

## Respiratory System

It is important to ascertain any factors that may be aggravating the client's ability to breathe easily. When assessing the status of the respiratory system, determination of activity pattern, as discussed in the client profile, is of prime importance. It is necessary to know to what extent respiratory changes incapacitate the individual. Respiratory diseases are more prevalent in the older person and questions regarding cough, sputum, and hemoptysis cannot be overlooked. The practitioner should keep in mind that, because the pain threshold is higher in older people, the experience of chest pain from pleuritis may be lessened or absent.

The lung is the most common site of cancer in males between 55 and 74 years of age and the second most common in males over 75 (Krumpe, Knudson, Parsons, & Reiser, 1985). A recurrent cough, fatigue, weight loss, shortness of breath, and sputum (at times bloody) are hallmarks of lung cancer. Presence of any combination of these signs and symptoms should be pursued vigorously.

There has been a resurgence in cases of tuberculosis in the elderly. Until recently, as many as 50% of cases of tuberculosis were in people 65 and over (Krumpe et al., 1985). Most of these cases are thought to be reactivation of long-dormant infections. Among the elderly, people 70 and over have the highest mortality rate from pulmonary tuberculosis. Reactivation of tuberculosis may be related to alterations in the immune and inflammatory response mechanisms with aging, as well as to nutritional deficiencies, excessive alcohol consumption, and glucocorticosteroid therapy. For these reasons the examiner should be particularly observant of weight loss, night sweats, or changes in respiratory status such as coughing.

## Hematopoietic System

Fatigue and weakness are among the most common complaints of the older person. These complaints are vague and can be the result of a variety of diseases. However, the possibility of anemia must always be considered in the older individual. Studies have documented the presence of anemia in 12% to 20% of the elderly (Timiras & Brownstein, 1987). Iron deficiency anemia is the most common type of anemia. While inadequate iron intake and altered gastrointestinal absorption of iron are often contributing factors, it is unlikely that one would become anemic as a result of these factors alone. The most common cause of anemia is gastrointestinal bleeding (Lewis, 1976). Therefore, it is important to obtain an explicit diet history and a history of any changes in bowel patterns or of melena.

The prevalence of Acquired Immune Deficiency Syndrome (AIDS) is relatively small in the elderly population; only 10% of all cases are in people aged 50 and over (Moss & Miles, 1987). It is necessary, however, to ask specific questions to assess risk. Such questions include history of blood transfusion before 1985, sexual contact with high risk individuals, or IV drug use.

# PHYSICAL EXAMINATION

## Cardiac System

Inspection, percussion, and palpation of the precordium of the normal older adult differ little from the examination of a normal younger adult. In the absence of disease, heart size remains the same throughout life. The apex of the heart may be displaced from its usual position due to kyphoscoliosis or obesity. Palpation of the PMI or heart contours may not be helpful in estimating heart size in the elderly.

Congestive heart failure is extremely common in the older adult. The examiner should observe and record baseline data related to the signs and symptoms of congestive heart failure (CHF).

Calcification or mucoid degeneration is responsible for degenerative valve disease in the elderly. Calcification is found in approximately 33% of patients 75 and over (Grawlinski & Jensen, 1991). On auscultation, extra sounds may be heard in the normal older person. As $S_4$ may be more commonly found but, in the absence of cardiovascular disease, the $S_4$ may be considered a normal variant of age (O'Rourke, Chatterjee, & Wei, 1987). A soft systolic ejection murmur, occurring early in systole and heard best at the base of the heart, may be heard in at least 20% of older clients and is considered innocent in the absence of signs or symptoms of cardiac disease. This systolic murmur is probably caused by aortic dilation or fusion of aortic valve commissures.

Cardiac output may not decrease in the healthy older adult, but activity tolerance is diminished. The examiner can test activity tolerance by checking the pulse rate prior to and following some physical exercise appropriate to the client's usual level of activity. Care should be taken when exercising to avoid levels beyond cardiac reserve. For example, in a client with limited reserve, the ability to move from a sitting to a standing position or to flex and extend fingers rapidly may be used to measure activity tolerance. The normal rise in pulse rate should be no greater than 10 to 20 beats per minute and should return to the basal or resting state within 2 minutes. The heart rate of the older client will increase but may not increase as much as a young person's and the pulse may take longer to return to its pre-exercise rate (Schulman & Gerstenblith, 1989). For definitive evaluation of activity tolerance, the client should be referred for stress testing under controlled conditions.

Blood pressure should be assessed in the sitting and lying positions. As a result of loss of elasticity in the aorta and arteries, blood pressure often increases with age. As many as 25% to 44% of persons over 50 years of age may have elevated blood pressures (Roberts & Rowlands, 1981). Blacks have a higher incidence of hypertension, with 44% reported for blacks and 33% for whites (Anderson, 1988). Both systolic and diastolic pressures rise with age, but there is a greater increase in the systolic pressure. This results in a widening of the pulse pressure.

Much controversy surrounds the definition of hypertension in the older person, but normal blood pressures are associated with increased longevity, and elevation of blood pressure is eventually associated with some degree of end organ damage. Increased morbidity has been associated with diastolic systolic hypertension (diastolic blood pressure over 90 mmHg) and recent studies show systolic blood pressure over 160 mmHg is also associated with increased morbidity in the elderly. Therefore, any person with documented blood pressure reading above 160/90 should receive follow-up.

With normal aging, a slight decrease in heart rate may be seen but, in the absence of disease, both heart rate and rhythm should be near normal. Older individuals respond less effectively to the stress of exercise, emotionally charged situations, and elevated temperature. The heart rate response is lower and a longer time is needed for the heart rate to return to baseline. It is difficult to differentiate the contribution made by age, disease, and cardiac conditioning to the functioning of the elderly heart. Older people tend not to remain physically active and cardiac deconditioning is common (LaKetta & Gerstenblith, 1990).

The elderly are prone to arrhythmias, even in the absence of overt cardiac disease. The sinus and atrioventricular nodes exhibit decreased size, infiltration with collagen and fat, amyloid deposits, and lipofuscin accumulation (Klausner & Schwartz, 1985). The number of pacemaker cells in the sinus node diminishes to roughly 10% of what is found in younger individuals, and the aging heart may experience as much as a 50% loss of fibers in the Bundle of His (Grawlinski & Jensen, 1991). In one study, 88% of healthy individuals between the ages of 60 and 85 had some form of ventricular or supraventricular arrhythmia in a 24-hour period (Fleg & Kennedy, 1982). Individuals with a transient tachycardia are more prone to heart failure. These arrhythmias may be the heralding feature of cardiac disease. As with any arrhythmia, the measurement of the apical and radial pulses are indicated to determine the presence of a pulse deficit.

## Vascular System

The pulses of all locations (carotid, brachial, radial, femoral, popliteal, posterior tibial, and dorsalis pedis) must be examined carefully. Blood vessels elongate and become more tortuous and prominent with advancing age. The arteries may be more firm due to arteriosclerotic change in the vessel walls. In some instances vessels may be easier to palpate due to loss of supportive surrounding tissues. On the other hand, the most distal lower extremity pulses may be more difficult to feel in the older client due to decreased arterial perfusion.

Assessment of the carotid pulses is especially important in the examination of older clients (see Figure 7.1). As for all clients, the examiner palpates only one carotid pulse at a time, since the cerebral perfusion may already be compromised and further diminution of blood flow may cause a syncopal attack or stroke. The pulse should be palpated gently to avoid stimulating the vagal receptors in the neck or dislodging any existing atherosclerotic plaques.

Auscultation for bruits in the carotid arteries should be an integral part of the examination. The presence of a bruit requires prompt follow-up because of the high risk for developing a cerebrovascular accident and because, in certain instances, endarterectomy may be warranted (North American Symptomatic Carotid Endarterectomy Trial Collaborators, 1991). The practitioner needs to differentiate bruits from the sound of cardiac murmurs radiating to the neck.

Assessment of the extremities includes evaluation of the older client's vascular status, both arterial and venous. The legs are more distal to

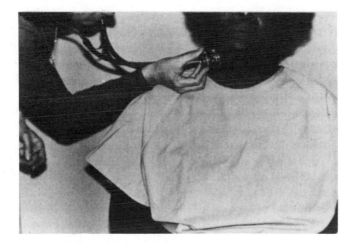

FIGURE 7.1 Assessment of the carotid pulse.

the heart and likely to be dependent and, therefore, the first location to show evidence of arterial and venous disease.

The presence of arterial insufficiency, most often associated with arteriosclerosis and diabetes mellitus, will result in a combination of the following physical findings: cool, thin, shiny, and taut skin; decreased hair distribution; thickened, brittle nails; gray pallor on elevation of the extremity; dusky mottled appearance when the leg is lowered (dependent rubor); and diminished or absent peripheral pulses. Hair loss occurs normally with advanced age and this alone is not a good indication of arterial insufficiency in the legs. The practitioner should be aware that the dorsalis pedis pulse is absent in approximately 20% of older people. Pulses proximal to the diminished or absent pulse need to be carefully assessed to pinpoint the level of arterial occlusion. The femoral arteries should be auscultated for bruits. A sequela of arterial disease is ulceration, which results from ischemia and trauma.

Stasis dermatitis and varicosities are evidence of venous disease common to an older population (see Figure 7.2). Varicosities are a problem only if cords, ulcerations, or signs of thrombophlebitis are present. Cords are nontender, palpable veins having a rubber tubing consistency. If varicosities are evident, their size and distribution should be noted. The skin over the ankle or lower calf may show evidence of scars of healed varicose ulcers and areas of patchy, brownish discoloration. On palpation, brawny, nonpitting edema may be elicited. If thrombophlebitis is suspected, inflammation can be determined by palpation of skin temperature and testing for the presence of Homan's sign.

The practitioner should determine the presence of lower extremity edema, a common finding in clients with congestive heart failure or venous insufficiency. Presence of pitting edema is determined by applying pressure over a bone of the foot, either at the instep (dorsum) or over the medial malleolus. If edema is present distally, one should assess further up on the leg for pretibial edema and sacral edema. Edema is evaluated as pitting or non-pitting and is graded trace, 1+, 2+, 3+, and 4+.

## Respiratory System

Examination of the exterior chest may reveal some common findings in the aged. Kyphosis, the accentuation of the thoracic curve, is caused by the osteoporotic collapse of vertebrae in the spinal column. The

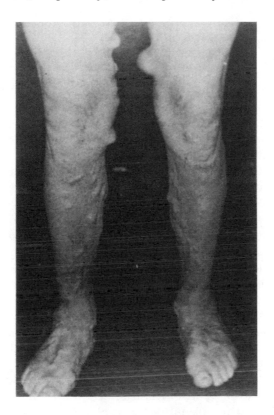

**FIGURE 7.2 Prominent bilateral varicose veins.**

From Rossman, I. 1971. *Clinical Geriatrics*. Philadelphia: J.B. Lippincott Co. Reprinted with permission.

change in the spine causes the individual to appear to be leaning forward. Upon palpation, the loss of vertebral bone may be palpated if compression fractures have occurred due to osteoporosis. If spinal scoliosis is present, the trachea may be deviated from the midline. The bony landmarks of the neck, ribs, and sternum may appear more prominent due to a loss of subcutaneous fat.

At times, a widening of the anterioposterior (A-P) distance of the chest is seen. This barrel-chest structural deformity is called senile emphysema but can be differentiated from the barrel-chest secondary to chronic obstructive lung disease by the absence of abnormal pulmonary findings on percussion and auscultation.

The quality, rhythm, and rate of quiet respirations are similar for the older and younger adult. Cheyne-Stokes respiration, that is, periods of apnea followed by deep breaths, may be observed as a normal variation when the older client is asleep.

In the normal aged adult, breathing rate and rhythm are unchanged at rest, but with exercise the rate will increase and take longer to return to pre-exercise rates. The dead space increases with advancing age and, concomitantly, the vital capacity decreases. The forced expiratory volume also decreases with age, and this change mimics minor airway obstruction. The older person may not have obstructive airway disease but continues to be at greater risk for cardiac or pulmonary disease (Wahba, 1983).

A decreased expansion of the rib cage may be caused by the loss of accessory musculature. This, along with increased lung rigidity ("stiff lungs"), causes a change in distribution of ventilation, specifically decreased air flow to the base and normal or increased air flow to the apex. Because of the loss of musculature, a diminished ability to cough forcefully may also be observed (Krumpe et al., 1985).

Rib fractures due to osteoporosis are more common in the older client. Even a slight blow or fall may cause an undetected fracture. The site of the fracture is easily found by eliciting point tenderness. This is done by holding one hand firmly on the anterior chest and the other hand firmly on the posterior chest. With each deep inspiration, pain will be elicited at the point of the fracture.

On percussion, the normal older adult's lungs sound resonant. If structural changes are present, such as kyphosis or senile emphysema, increased resonance may be elicited over the affected areas. If pneumonia is present, a common problem with the older adult, hyperresonance or dullness may be found over the areas of consolidation.

Auscultatory sounds over the normal lung are the same for the younger and older adult. Vesicular breath sounds should be audible throughout the lung fields. Since lung expansion may be diminished, the examiner may need to re-emphasize the necessity of taking deep breaths with the mouth open. If structural deformities such as kyphosis or senile emphysema are present, breath sounds may be distant over those areas. Rales or rhonci are heard only in the presence of disease.

## Hematopoietic System

Blood dyscrasias are not normally more prevalent in the older adult population. The nurse should look for the common signs of anemia by noting the color of nail beds, conjunctiva, and buccal mucosa. However, Schouten (1975) advises that inspection of the hands gives a better indication of the hemoglobin level in the older client than inspection of the conjunctiva. If the normal red lines are apparent in the folds of the palms when the hand is slightly stretched, anemia is unlikely. If pale palm lines are seen, the hemoglobin may be less than half normal value (Schouten, 1975). Laboratory reports are necessary to confirm this finding.

## NURSING IMPLICATIONS

The complete data base helps the nurse in formulating plans and is needed to determine if the findings are age or disease related. For example, a systolic ejection murmur needs to be documented for later reference, should the client develop cardiac disease.

It is important to include health promotional teaching (see Appendix). The healthy (or not so healthy) older person should be advised to stop smoking and to maintain a regular exercise regimen. Reducing risk for cardiovascular and respiratory disease may require substantial changes in habits and lifestyle. The stereotype that older people have lived their lives and are unable to change speaks against the belief that all people, young and old, should be provided with the necessary information to select among available options for self-management of their health care. Individuals should plan a form of daily exercise. Diet should include a variety of foods in the amounts suggested in the Food Guide Pyramid (see Chapter 8). Older people should avoid contact with individuals with upper respiratory infections. These are the types of lifestyle modifications which will help to reduce the risk of developing cardiac and respiratory disease.

Respiratory infection is common in the older adult. Decreased ability of the bronchial cilia to clear foreign matter, decreased immunologic responses, and decreased lung capacity combine to make the older individual more susceptible. The number of and pattern of response to respiratory infections will guide the practitioner in further assessment data and in planning for care. Because there is an increased susceptibility to lower respiratory tract infections, it is particularly important with the elderly to determine the history of immunization against influenza, which should be done annually. Similarly, older people should receive vaccination against pneumococcal pneumonia once every 10 years.

Activity usually does not need to be specifically restricted, because fatigue and shortness of breath will act to limit exercise. Therefore, the statement, "You need to watch your exercise," should not be made before a complete exercise history is documented and a total assessment of exercise capabilities is made.

The individual who experiences dizziness upon rising, should be advised to rise slowly. Placing the telephone near the bed or couch, or advising family members to allow the phone to ring for long times, may help to diminish the need to rise quickly.

Because of the high incidence of peripheral vascular disease, the practitioner should be aware of the need for preventive care. The client should be taught to examine his or her feet for signs of trauma or skin breakdown. The feet should be kept clean, dry, and well lubricated. The older client should be advised to wear cotton socks and avoid restrictive clothing. If foot or nail deformities are present, the areas should be padded with lambs' wool and holes put in the shoes if necessary. A home visit may reveal sources of potential trauma, such as low furniture, which may cause injury to the feet and legs, or pets, who may scratch the legs.

## REFERENCES

Anderson, S. (1988). Aging and hypertension among elderly blacks. Jackson, J. (Ed.), *The black American elderly*. New York: Springer Publishing Co.

Fleg, J. L., & Kennedy, H. L. (1982). Cardiac arrhythmias in a healthy elderly population. Detection by 24-hour ambulatory electrocardiography. *Chest, 81*(3), 302–307.

Grawlinski, A., & Jensen, G. (1991). The complications of cardiovascular aging. *American Journal of Nursing 91*(11), 26–30.

Halperin, J. L. (1987). Peripheral vascular disease: Medical evaluation and treatment. *Geriatrics, 42*(11), 47–61.

Kannel, W. B., Dannenberg, A. L., & Abbott, R. D. (1985). Unrecognized myocardial infarction and hypertension: The Framingham Study. *American Heart Journal, 109*(3), 581–585.

Klausner, S. C., & Schwartz, A. B. (1985). The aging heart. *Clinics in Geriatric Medicine, 1*(1), 119–141.

Krumpe, P. E., Knudson, R. J., Parsons, G., & Reiser, K. (1985). The aging respiratory system. *Clinics in Geriatric Medicine, 1*(1), 143–175.

LaKetta, E. G., & Gerstenblith, G. (1990). Alterations in circulatory function. In Hazzard, W. R., Andres, R., Bierman, E. L., & Blass, J. P. (Eds.), *Principles of geriatric medicine and gerontology*. New York: McGraw-Hill, Inc.

Lewis, R. (1976). Anemia—a common but never normal concomitant of aging. *Geriatrics, 31*(12), 53–60.

Lipsitz, L. A. (1989). Orthostatic hypotension in the elderly. *New England Journal of Medicine, 321*(14), 952–957.

Moss, R. J., & Miles, S. H. (1987). AIDS and the geriatrician. *Journal of the American Geriatrics Society, 35*(5), 460–464.

National Center for Health Statistics. Havlik, R. J. et al. (1987). Health statistics on older persons. *Vital and Health Statistics*, (series 3, No. 24). Washington, DC: U.S. Government Printing Office.

North American Symptomatic Carotid Endarteretomy Trial Collaborators. (1991). Beneficial effect of carotid endarterectomy in symptomatic patients with high-grade carotid stenosis. *New England Journal of Medicine, 325*, 446–453.

O'Rourke, R. A., Chatterjee, K., & Wei, J. Y. (1987). Coronary heart disease. *Journal of the American College of Cardiology, 10*(2), 52A–56A.

Roberts, J., & Rowland, M. (1981). Hypertension in adults 25–74 years of age. *Vital and Health Statistics* (Series 11, No. 221). Washington, DC: U.S. Government Printing Office.

Schouten, J. (1975). Important factors in the examination and care of old patients. *Journal of the American Geriatrics Society, 23*(4), 180–183.

Schulman, S. P., & Gerstenblith, G. (1989). Cardiovascular changes with aging. The response to exercise. *Journal of Cardiopulmonary Rehabilitation, 9*(1), 12–16.

SHEP Cooperative Research Group. (1991). Prevention of stroke by antihypertensive drug treatment in older persons with Isolated systolic hypertension. *Journal of the American Medical Association, 265*(24), 3255–3264

Smith, D. A., Karmally, W., & Brown, W. V. (1987). Treating hyperlipidemia part 1: Whether and when in the elderly. *Geriatrics, 42*(6), 33–44.

Timiras, M. L., & Brownstein, H. (1987). Prevalence of anemia and corre-lation of hemoglobin with age in a geriatric screening clinic population. *Journal of the American Geriatrics Society, 35*(7), 639–643.

Wahba, W. M. (1983). Influence of aging on lung function—clinical signi-ficances of changes from age twenty. *Anesthesia and Analgesia, 62*(8), 764–776.

# SUGGESTED READINGS

Cassel, C. K., Riesenberg, D. E., Sorensen, L. B., & Walsh, J. R. ed. (1990). *Geriatric Medicine*. New York: Springer-Verlag.

Gerber, R. M. (1990). Coronary artery disease in the elderly. *The Journal of Cardio-vascular Nursing, 4*(4), 23–34.

The 1988 report of the Joint National Committee on detection, evaluation, and treatment of high blood pressure. (1988). *Archives of Internal Medicine, 148*(5), 1023–1038.

Rebenson-Piano, M. (1989, June). The physiologic changes that occur with aging. *Critical Care Quarterly, 12*(1), 1–14.

Sowers, J. R. (1987, January 26). Hypertension in the elderly. *American Journal of Medicine, 82*(Suppl. 1B), 1–8.

Walsh, R. A. (1987, Jan. 26). Cardiovascular effects of the aging process. *The American Journal of Medicine, 82*(Suppl. 1B), 34–40.

# 8

# Assessment of Nutritional Status, Gastrointestinal Functioning, and Abdominal Examination

## PAST HEALTH HISTORY

### Nutrition

Nutritional status has been implicated in the health and well-being of the elderly. Dietary intake can influence the onset of illness such as cardiovascular disease, or complicate existing disease such as diabetes mellitus.

Malnutrition has been found in as many as 61% of individuals 65 years of age and over hospitalized in a Veterans Administration Hospital (Bienia, Ratcliff, Barbour et al., 1989). Nurses do not use the full array of indicators of malnutrition available to them. Researchers have found 40% more patients malnourished than were assessed to be malnourished by staff nurses (Collinsworth & Boyle, 1989).

Nutrition screening is used to determine individuals with actual and/ or the potential for malnutrition. The most important aspect of assessment is the nutritional history. Recall of food and beverage intake for a 24-hour period is difficult in the best of circumstances, and poses a real challenge with the elderly. The practitioner should ask the client to relate the full intake for the past 24 hours in his or her own words. The practitioner can then supplement the nutritional picture by asking questions regarding preparation of food and use of condiments and vitamin supplements. Approximately 37% of adults, often individuals least in need, take a food supplement (Kaplan, Annest, Layda et al., 1986). Table 8.1 shows the Recommended Daily Allowance (RDA) for males and females 51 years of age and older. A quick way to assess for nutritional intake is to determine whether the individual eats the variety of foods as shown in the Food Guide Pyramid shown in Table 8.2. The Food Guide Pyramid emphasizes the quantity of foods appropriate to each of the five food groups. If one area is consumed to a disproportionate level, either more or less food, the individual may be at risk for specific health problems. The individual, for example, who consumes no dairy products is at risk for osteoporosis. The individual who greatly restricts protein intake may have poor healing capabilities. A low protein intake, combined with the emotional and physical stress of chronic disease, makes the older individual more vulnerable to infections and protein deficiency.

**TABLE 8.1 Recommended Daily Allowance (RDA) for Individuals 51 Years of Age and Older**

|                        | Male  | Female |
|------------------------|-------|--------|
| Vitamin A (µg RE)      | 1,000 | 800    |
| Vitamin D (µg)         | 5     | 5      |
| Vitamin E (mg α-TE)    | 10    | 8      |
| Vitamin K (µg)         | 80    | 65     |
| Vitamin C (mg)         | 60    | 60     |
| Thiamin (mg)           | 1.2   | 1.0    |
| Riboflavin (mg)        | 1.4   | 1.2    |
| Niacin (mg NE)         | 15    | 13     |
| Vitamin $B_6$ (mg)     | 2.0   | 1.6    |
| Folate (µg)            | 200   | 180    |
| Vitamin $B_{12}$ (µg)  | 2.0   | 2.0    |
| Calcium (mg)           | 800   | 800    |
| Phosphorus (mg)        | 800   | 800    |
| Magnesium (mg)         | 350   | 280    |
| Iron (mg)              | 10    | 10     |
| Zinc (mg)              | 15    | 12     |
| Iodine (µg)            | 150   | 150    |
| Selenium (µg)          | 70    | 55     |

Reprinted with permission from *Recommended Dietary Allowances*, © 1989 by The National Academy of Sciences. Published by National Academy Press, Washington, DC.

**TABLE 8.2 Food Guide Pyramid**

# Now, 5 Food Groups

The Federal Government has adapted the Food Guide Pyramid as its primary device for educating the public about nutrition.

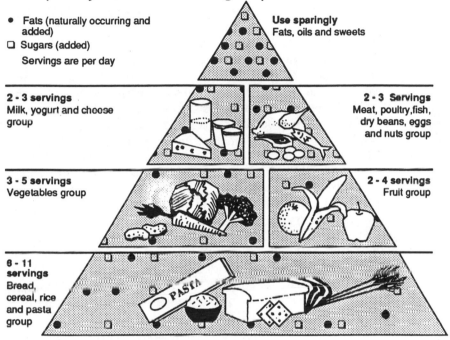

- Fats (naturally occurring and added)
- Sugars (added)

Servings are per day

**Use sparingly**
Fats, oils and sweets

**2 - 3 servings**
Milk, yogurt and choose group

**2 - 3 Servings**
Meat, poultry, fish, dry beans, eggs and nuts group

**3 - 5 servings**
Vegetables group

**2 - 4 servings**
Fruit group

**6 - 11 servings**
Bread, cereal, rice and pasta group

*Source: U.S. Department of Agriculture*

Knowledge of cultural preferences can enhance the practitioner's ability to ask pointed questions. Individuals of Hispanic origin may fry foods in palm oil, high in cholesterol, while individuals of Oriental descent may use large quantities of MSG, high in sodium content.

A history of the social context of food and eating will provide data concerning the meaning of meals to the older individual. Has the client always eaten with family members and now eats alone? Has the older client's preparation of meals for the family been a way of giving to loved ones which is now lost?

Questions regarding changes in patterns of eating are important. In what ways is the diet different today than it was 10 years ago? or 3 months ago? What has contributed to the change: Is it financial or loss of a spouse? Does the client eat more canned or processed foods when only fresh fruits and vegetables were once eaten? Canned and processed foods are often high in sodium and do not provide the dietary fiber found in fresh fruits and vegetables. In extreme cases older individuals may even be found to eat food scraps or pet food. Individuals may eat infrequently or only one meal a day. The practitioner needs to keep an open mind to possible variations in eating patterns.

Physical impairments may impact on nutrition. Has vision diminished to a point where the individual cannot see to cook or shop? Has hearing diminished so that it is difficult to attend a nutrition center? Is there difficulty chewing or swallowing food?

Weight patterns and caloric intake are important to determine. Caloric need decreases with age. As individuals become older, the level of physical activity diminishes, lean body mass decreases, and the basal metabolic rate (BMR) lowers. Obesity is a problem for many older people. Generally, individuals 65 and over need to restrict daily intake to between 1280 to 1900 calories for females and between 1530 to 2300 calories for males (National Research Council Recommended Dietary Allowances, 1989). Within each range the number of calories ingested should be moderated by the degree of physical activity, with a lower number of calories for sedentary individuals and a higher number for active individuals. Older people who follow weight reduction diets risk developing malnutrition, vitamin deficiencies, or anemias. It is important to determine milk consumption, a common source of calcium and Vitamin D, as osteoporosis is common in older adults, particularly women. One third of women over 65 will experience vertebral and hip fractures due to bone demineralization (National Research Council, 1989).

Sensory deficits, such as diminished sense of smell, may make food less palatable. The use of sweets, spices, and condiments may be exaggerated to compensate for otherwise "tasteless" food. Because of the high incidence of congestive heart failure in older people, the amount of salt used in cooking, added at the table, and ingested in such foods as smoked meats, prepared foods, or condiments must be carefully ascertained.

It is particularly important to determine the older client's pattern of fluid intake in order to assess fluid and electrolyte balance. A daily intake of at least 1,300 cc of fluid is recommended. In general, older adults have a decreased thirst and a diminished total fluid intake. Medications commonly prescribed for older people, such as diuretics, tend to further deplete fluid reserves. For some older people, such as clients with congestive heart failure, fluid intake may need to be curtailed.

Excessive gas, or flatulence, and constipation are two commonly reported problems. The practitioner should determine if gas-producing foods are eaten, as well as estimate the fiber content in the diet. The elderly specifically need to be asked questions regarding how they avoid and treat constipation. Is there a pattern of nutritional supplements, for example, prunes or bran, or is there a medical regimen, for example, stool softeners or laxatives?

A complete drug history may reveal the use of medications which alter fluid, electrolyte, and nutritional status. Overuse of medications and polypharmacy present a challenge to the practitioner. Unfortunately, there is a paucity of literature about the full extent of nutrient loss complicated by medication buildup and/or changes in fat and lean body mass. Table 8.3 presents a list of drugs commonly taken by older

**TABLE 8.3 Drug–Nutrient Interaction**

| Medication | Potential effect on nutrients |
| --- | --- |
| mineral oil | reduces absorption of fat-soluble vitamins A, D, E, and K |
| anticonvulsants | reduces storage of vitamin K and absorption of calcium and vitamin D |
| antacids containing aluminum | reduces absorption of phosphorus and fluoride and raises excretion of calcium |
| antacids containing aluminum or magnesium | reduces absorption and raises intestinal elimination of phosphate |
| antacids containing sodium-bicarbonate | causes sodium overload and water retention |
| gentamicin | raises potassium and magnesium excretion |
| penicillin | raises potassium excretion |
| tetracyclines | reduces absorption of iron, calcium, zinc, and magnesium |
| aspirin | reduces serum levels of folate and ascorbic acid, causes iron deficiency secondary to blood loss |
| corticosteroids | reduces calcium and phosphorus absorption, raises the need for pyridoxine, folate, ascorbic acid, and vitamin D |
| potassium supplements | reduces absorption of vitamin $B_{12}$ secondary to diminished acidity in the ileum |
| laxatives | causes hypokalemia, hypoalbuminemia, lower calcium absorption, malabsorption with steatorrhea |
| cholestyramine | reduces absorption of fat-soluble vitamins and calcium |
| cimetidine | reduces absorption of vitamin $B_{12}$ as a result of hypochlorhydria |
| neomycin | reduces absorption of fat, lactose, nitrogen, calcium, iron, potassium, and vitamin $B_{12}$ |
| Isoniazid | causes vitamin $B_6$ and niacin deficiency |
| Hydralazine | causes vitamin $B_6$ deficiency |

*Note.* Miller, C. (1990, Dec.). When medication harms as well as helps. *Geriatric Nursing,* *11*(6), 301–302. Used with permission.

people and their potential effect on nutrient absorption, utilization and/ or secretion. Table 8.4 lists drugs with documented side effects on the gastrointestinal tract. Intake of foods may alter the absorption and excretion of certain medications and is a particular concern when the drug has a narrow therapeutic range, for example, propranolol or dicumarol (Pinto, 1991).

# PAST HEALTH HISTORY

## Gastrointestinal System

Dysphagia (difficulty swallowing) is a common complaint of the elderly and is potentially quite serious if, for example, the cause is a tumor or stricture. It is important to differentiate between real difficulty in swallowing and regurgitation or "heartburn." Questions concerning food getting "stuck in the throat" or the ease with which solid versus liquid food can be swallowed will help in clarifying symptoms. Difficulty swallowing can be terribly frightening to clients. Slowed or disorganized esophageal motility can occur in the aged person (presbyesophagus). If severe, it can cause discomfort as the food passes through the esophagus.

**TABLE 8.4 Drugs with Gastrointestinal Side Effects**

| Medications | Possible adverse reactions |
| --- | --- |
| lithium, chlorpromazine, phenothiazines, diazepine, cyproheptadine | stimulate appetite |
| digoxin, theophylline, antihistamines, over-the-counter cold or sleep preparations | anorexia |
| narcotics, psychotropic medications, aluminum hydroxide calcium carbonate, anticholinergics | constipation |
| cimetidine, propranolol, laxatives, clindamycin; antacids containing magnesium hydroxide | diarrhea |
| loop and thiazide diuretis, antipsychotics (especially phenothiazines), antidepressants, ß sympathomimetics, antihistamines, decongestants, anticholinergics | dry mouth |
| ibuprofen, phenylbutazone, indomethacin, sallcylates, phenobarbital, corticosteroids | gastric irritation |
| furosemide and other potassium-depleting medications, anticholinergics | paralytic ileus |
| bulk-forming agents taken before meals | early satiety |

Adapted from Miller, C. (1990, Dec.). When medication harms as well as helps. *Geriatric Nursing 11*(6), 301–302. Used with permission.

Although food intolerance is a common complaint of the elderly, there seems to be little biologic reason for the complaint in the absence of disease. The gastric production of hydrochloric acid does decrease with age, but, in the absence of disease, this causes no problem. Hiatal hernia is another common problem. While only 9% of people over 40 years old have hiatal hernias, the incidence increases to 69% in people over 70 years of age (Hyams, 1974). A careful history of food intake that reveals substernal pain or discomfort after eating, or discomfort when lying flat after eating or at night, suggests the presence of hiatal hernia with esophageal reflux. Often the older individual will state a preference for eating the evening meal at 5:00 or 6:00 p.m. A commonly heard complaint is "I just don't sleep well if I eat meals late at night." A hiatal hernia may be the underlying cause of the discomfort following late night food ingestion.

It is sometimes difficult to determine the difference between pain of cardiac or gastrointestinal origin. Pain in the chest is potentially cardiac in origin and potentially life threatening. A thorough exploration of pain in the chest or abdomen is indicated as substernal chest discomfort may be gastrointestinal rather than cardiac. Table 8.5 presents a comparison of pain symptoms seen with cardiac and gastrointestinal disease. The comparison can help to differentiate the source of the discomfort.

The practitioner should remember that pain may not always be reported when gastrointestinal problems are present. The pain threshold in the elderly is often elevated; thus, major abdominal pathology, such as appendicitis or acute abdomen, may go undetected.

Table 8.6 indicates the types of cancers prevalent in older age groups (ranked in order of incidence by sex). Colon and rectal cancer are among the three most frequent sites of cancer for both males and females over 55 years of age. The incidence of colorectal cancer increases with a family history. Therefore, the family history is important. Individuals with a past history of polyps, adenomas, or inflammatory bowel disease are also at a higher risk for developing colorectal cancer in older age. A history of weight loss, change in bowel habits, and rectal bleeding should alert the practitioner to the possibility of this type of malignancy.

Constipation is a frequent complaint of the older client. Constipation may be defined as too few bowel movements, excessively hard, dry feces, or lack of a feeling of clearance or relief after a bowel movement. Constipation is not normal and should be fully explored. A recent change in bowel habits may indicate an acute process. The practitioner needs to obtain a careful description of the character and number of stools per week.

**TABLE 8.5 Comparison of Pain of Cardiac and Gastrointestinal Origin**

| Pain characteristic | Cardiac origin | Gastrointestinal origin |
|---|---|---|
| Description | Usually tightness, but can be any type of pain | Usually burning or fullness, but can be any type of pain |
| Location | Usually in chest | May be in chest or abdomen |
| Radiation | Radiation occurs commonly down the left arm, but can be to neck or jaw | Ulcer pain usually radiates to the back Gallbladder pain usually radiates to right shoulder |
| Onset | Usually rapid | Usually rapid |
| Duration | Anginal pain disappears in 10 to 15 minutes Infarction pain can persist | Can be of long or short duration |
| Aggravating factors | Activity or anxiety Anginal pain relieved by nitroglycerin | Related to food; either to ingestion or lack of food intake |
| Relieving factors | Rest Anginal pain relieved by nitroglycerin | May be relieved by antacids, food, or upright position Not relieved by nitroglycerine |

**TABLE 8.6 Deaths from Cancer in Older Age Groups**

| Most frequent sites age 55 to 74 | | Most frequent sites age 75–84 | | Most frequent sites age 85 & over | |
|---|---|---|---|---|---|
| Males | Females | Males | Females | Males | Females |
| Trachea, bronchus & lung | Trachea, bronchus & lung | Trachea, bronchus & lung | Trachea, bronchus & lung | Prostate | Breast |
| Prostate | Colon | Prostate | Breast | Trachea, bronchus & lung | Colon |
| Colon | Uterus | Colon | Colon | Colon | Trachea, bronchus & lung |
| Pancreas | | Pancreas | Pancreas | Bladder | Pancreas |

Source: National Center for Health Statistics. (1990). *Vital Statistics of the United States, 1988*, Vol II Mortality, Part B. DHHS Pub. No (PHS) 90-1102. Public Health Service, Washington, DC: U.S. Government Printing Office.

Constipation may have multiple etiologic factors related to the aging process. The transit time for stool to pass through the gastrointestinal tract is slowed resulting in increased reabsorption of water and harder stools. In addition, perception of sensory stimuli that produce the urge to defecate is diminished. Client-induced constipation can be caused by a combination of the following factors: lack of bulk foods in the diet, diminished fluid intake, diminished physical activity, a break in normal routine, chronic laxative ingestion, and a blunting or loss of the urge to defecate as a result of chronic denial of the urge. Iatrogenically induced constipation can result from the use of medications such as sedatives, tranquilizers, anticholinergics, antidepressants, opiates, or aluminum compounds (Maalox). A careful history of each of these etiological factors needs to be obtained to determine if the constipation is amenable to therapy.

The most severe form of constipation is fecal impaction. Here again, a detailed history of bowel habits needs to be obtained. The first sign of fecal impaction is often uncontrollable diarrhea or leakage of stool around the impaction. Fecal impaction is a potentially serious problem and early detection is important.

Fecal incontinence most often is a problem of the confused or neurologically impaired older person. Rectal sensation and tone are diminished and defecation may occur before the client is aware of the need to defecate or can reach the bathroom. Fecal incontinence could be due to functional impairment or environmental constraints, thus, it is important to identify the factors contributing to the problem. Between 30% to 33% of death certificates in the elderly list diarrhea as a contributing cause of death (Hyams, 1974). The older person experiencing diarrhea may quickly become dehydrated. The complaint of diarrhea should be followed up quickly (Lew, Glass, Gangarosa et al., 1991).

The liver, gallbladder, and pancreas change minimally with age. In the absence of disease, these changes produce no symptomatic manifestations.

## Abdominal Examination

The abdominal examination in the healthy older person should reveal nothing abnormal. The liver, pancreas, and kidneys normally decrease slightly in size, but this decrease is probably not appreciable on palpation or percussion. The abdomen may feel very soft because of the loss of abdominal musculature; therefore, underlying organs may be more easily palpated. The bladder is usually not palpable, but asymptomatic over-distention may be found in older individuals due to decreased sensory function or to confusion.

The rectal exam should never be omitted in the older person because masses are often low enough in the rectum to be palpated by the examining finger. If the client has severe arthritis, the knee-chest position may be very painful and impossible for the client to assume. A modification to a side-lying position may be necessary for comfort. Rectal tone may be diminished with age and the sensations produced by the insertion of the finger may be diminished. A test for occult blood is important after each rectal exam to ascertain if there is a small, undetected, gastrointestinal bleed, as from a silent gastrointestinal ulceration or cancer.

If the client is impacted, there may be blood around the stool following disimpaction because of the localized trauma caused by the procedure. A test for occult blood in the center of the disimpacted stool will help to ascertain whether the bleeding is from a source higher in the gastrointestinal tract or due to local trauma from the digital exam and disimpaction. In the client with fecal incontinence, the tone of the rectal sphincter will give some indication of the client's potential ability to regain continence.

## LABORATORY VALUES AS INDICATIONS OF NUTRITIONAL STATUS

Laboratory tests are available which provide an indication of nutritional status. (For a complete discussion of laboratory values, including normal values, see Chapter 14). Several tests relate directly to protein status. The most commonly utilized tests are total serum protein and serum albumin. Prealbumin, retinol binding protein, and transferrin are good indicators of protein status but are expensive and are used mainly to monitor individuals who have severe protein depletion. Very low serum albumin levels are associated with rapid decline and death in the elderly. Individuals with a deficit serum protein level will be more likely to have a problem with tissue regeneration, infections, fatigue, and immune deficiencies (Morley, 1990).

The range of normal vitamin levels is summarized in Table 8.7. Of these, the most frequently assessed are Vitamins A, D, K, $B_1$ (thiamine), $B_6$ (pyridoxide), $B_{12}$, and folic acid. Vitamins D, $B_6$, and $B_{12}$ have been found to be more likely to be deficient in the elderly where the deficiency is related to nutritional intake (Dwyer, 1989). Excessive amounts of the fat soluble vitamins (A, D, E, and K) can be life-threatening, as these vitamins are retained in fat stores.

**TABLE 8.7 Laboratory Tests for Assessment of Vitamin Status**

| Vitamin | Test | Unit of measure | Deficient | acceptable |
|---|---|---|---|---|
| Fat soluble | | | | |
| A | Serum vitamin A | µg/dL | < 20 | 15-60 |
| D | 25-hydroxy vitamin D | ng/mL | < 5 | 18-36 |
| | 1,25-dihydroxy vitamin D | pg/mL | | 22-40 |
| E | Plasma tocopherol | mg/dL | < .5 | > 0.5 |
| | Erythrocyte $H_2O_2$ hemolysis | percent | > 20 | < 5 |
| K | Prothrombin time | seconds | > 14 | 10 |
| Water soluble | | | | |
| $B_1$ (Thiamin) | Urinary excretion of Thiamin | µg/g thiamin/g creatinine | < 27 | ≥ 66 |
| $B_2$ (Riboflavin) | Urinary excretion of Riboflavin | µg/g creatinine | < 27 | ≥ 80 |
| | Erythrocyte glutathione reductase | A/C | > 1.4 | 1.0-1.2 |
| $B_3$ (Niacin) | Urinary excretion of N-methylnicotinamide | Excretion ratio of pyridone to methyl- nicotinamide | < 1.0 | 1.3-4.0 |
| $B_6$ (Pyridoxine) | Urinary excretion of Xanthurenic acid | mg/d | 25 | < 25 |
| Folic acid | Serum acid | ng/ml | < 3.0 | 5-16 |
| | Red blood cell folate | ng/mL | < 140 | ≥ 160 |
| $B_{12}$ | Serum $B_{12}$ | pg/mL | < 100 | 200-950 |
| C (ascorbic acid) | Plasma ascorbic acid | mg/dL | < .20 | 0.6-1.6 |

(See Henry, 1991; Shils & Young, 1988).

The laboratory tests that indicate nutritional status are also influenced by underlying disease status. Evaluation of individual laboratory tests needs to be completed in conjunction with any underlying physiologic problem.

Normal levels of the elements shown in Table 8.8 are necessary for maintaining a variety of bodily functions. Deficiencies of these elements may be seen in older individuals who have an inadequate diet. Although low iron is common in the elderly, it is rarely related to nutritional intake (Dwyer, 1989). Older individuals, particularly women, have bone demineralization. Calcium is one of the elements most likely to be deficient (Dwyer, 1989). Low serum levels of calcium may contribute to the escape of calcium from the bones.

**TABLE 8.8 Laboratory Tests of Assessment of the Elements**

| Element | Test | Unit of Measure | Deficient | Acceptable |
|---------|------|-----------------|-----------|------------|
| Calcium | serum calcium | mg/dL | < 8 | 8.4-10.2 |
| Iron | serum iron | µg/dL | < 60 | 60-150 |
| Magnesium | serum magnesium | mg/dL | | 1.8-3.0 |
| Phosphorus | serum phosphorus | mg/dL | <2 | 2.5-4.4 |
| Zinc | serum zinc | µg/dL | | 50-150 |

See Henry, 1991; Shils & Young, 1989).

# NURSING MEASURES

Following assessment of the dietary intake, the practitioner determines whether the individual is ingesting too little or an excess of the appropriate foods. The goal is to assist the individual to approach normal weight with the intake of a well-balanced diet.

For the overweight individual, incremental weekly changes can be made to decrease calorie intake utilizing the person's own dietary pattern. Weight should not be lost too rapidly, as people who lose weight rapidly tend to regain the weight. It is better to lose a pound or half-pound over a longer period of time than to lose weight rapidly. The practitioner needs to recommend a diet that slowly reduces caloric intake, coupled with an increase in physical exercise. The diet should be low in fats and sweets. (For recommendations regarding cholesterol intake, see Chapter 7). The health benefits of a low-fat diet are great. Sweet foods and foods high in fat have more calories per serving. A person can consume a larger amount and variety of foods if the foods are lower in calories. The hallmark of a good diet is a balance of the food groups according to the Food Guide Pyramid, coupled with ingestion of a variety of foods.

When the older individual is unable or not interested in eating, foods with higher nutrient density should be recommended. Chicken or fish have more protein per serving than peanut butter. Likewise, orange juice may be easier to ingest than a whole orange.

Recognizing that food is important in maintaining health, older people are particularly susceptible to food faddism. Many fad diets promise to increase longevity, improve health, and cure disease. These diets may, however, result in vitamin and/or mineral inadequacies or excesses. Diets that may be safe for younger adults may be detrimental to older clients. For example, a high-protein weight reduction diet, which promotes ketosis, may be harmful to older clients who have age-associated diminished renal function.

Often laboratory tests indicating nutritional status are available because the test is part of a series obtained for a primary health problem. The tests can be analyzed as a reflection of nutritional status, taking into account that the underlying disease state, rather than nutritional status, may cause the altered value.

Given the high incidence of bowel cancer in the elderly, and that occult or frank blood in the stool is an early symptom, testing for fecal blood loss is a major health objective for the elderly (U.S. Department of Health and Human Services, 1991). The target is for 50% of people 50 and older to have received fecal occult blood testing within the preceding 1 to 2 years, and to increase to at least 40% those who have ever received proctosigmoidoscopy. (See Appendix for other health promotion recommendations.)

## REFERENCES

Bienia, R., Ratcliff, S., Barbour, G. L., & Kummer, M. (1982). Malnutrition in the hospitalized geriatric patient. *Journal of the American Geriatrics Society*, *30*(7), 433–436.

Collinsworth, R., & Boyle, K. (1989). Nutritional assessment of the elderly. *Journal of Gerontological Nursing*, *15*(12), 17–21.

Dwyer, J. T. (1989). Screening older American's nutritional health: Current practices and future possibilities. Washington, DC. Department of Health and Human Sciences.

Henry, J. B. (1991). *Clinical diagnosis and management by laboratory methods*. Philadelphia: W.B. Saunders Co.

Hyams, D. E. (1974). Gastrointestinal problems in the old. *British Medical Journal*, *1*, 107–110.

Koplan, J. P., Annest, J. L., Layda, P. M., & Rubin, M. B. (1986). Nutrient intake and supplementation in the United States (NHANES II). *American Journal of Public Health*, *76*(3), 287–289.

Lew, J. F., Glass, R. I., Gangarosa, R. E. et al. (1991). Diarrheal deaths in the United States, 1979 through 1987. *Journal of the American Medical Association*, *265*(24), 3280–3284.

Morley, J. E. (1990). Nutrition and aging. In Hazzard, W. R., Andres, R., Bierman, E. L., & Blass, J. P. (Eds.), *Principles of geriatric medicine and gerontology*. New York: McGraw-Hill, Inc.

National Research Council. (1989). *Diet and health: Implications for reducing chronic disease risk*. Washington, DC: National Academy Press.

National Research Council. (1989). *Recommended dietary allowances*, 10th ed. Washington, DC: National Academy Press.

Pinto, J. T. (1991). The pharmacokinetic and pharmacodynamic inter-actions of food and drugs. *Topics in Clinical Nutrition*, *6*(3), 14–33.

Shils, M. E., & Young, V. R. (1988). *Modern nutrition in health and disease*. Philadelphia: Lea & Febiger.

U.S. Department of Health and Human Services. (1991). *Healthy people 2000: National health promotion and disease prevention.* Rockville, MD: Public Health Service.

# SUGGESTED READINGS

Collinsworth, R., & Boyle, K. (1985). Nutritional assessment of the elderly. *Journal of Gerontological Nursing, 15*(12), 17–21.

Hazzard, W. R., Andres, R., Bierman, E. L., & Blass, J. P. (Eds.). (1990). *Principles of geriatric medicine and gerontology.* New York: McGraw-Hill, Inc.

Hess, L. V. (1989). Nutritional care of the geriatric patient. *Journal of Home Health Care Practice, 2*(1), 29–38.

Nestle, M., & Gilbride, J. A. (1990). Nutrition policies for health promotion in older adults: Education priorities for the 1990's. *Journal of Nutrition Education, 22*(6), 314–317.

Weinrich, S. P., Blesch, K. S., Dickson, G. W., Nussbaum, J. S., & Watson, E. J. (1989). Timely detection of colorectal cancer in the elderly: Implications of the aging process. *Cancer Nursing, 12*(3), 170–176.

Weinrich, S. P., Blesch, K. S., Dickson, G. W., Nussbaum, J. S., & Watson, E. J. (1987). Position of the American Dietetic Association: Issues in feeding the terminally ill adult. *Journal of the American Dietetic Association, 87*(1), 78–85.

White, J. V., Ham, R. J., Lipschitz, D. A., Dwyer, J. T., & Wellman, N. S. (1991). Consensus of the nutrition screening initiative: risk factors and indicators of poor nutritional status in older Americans. *Journal of the American Dietetic Association, 91*(7), 783–787.

# 9

# Assessment of Sexual, Genital, and Urinary Functioning

## HISTORY

### Client Profile

The client profile will reveal important data relevant to the breast, sexual, genital, and urinary assessment. The practitioner needs a clear description of the client's home setting, including the number of rooms, the location of the kitchen and bathroom, and whether there are stairs to the bedroom, bathroom, or outside.

The status of significant relationships is important. Questions should determine who lives in the home with the client and who, if anyone, visits the client regularly. The practitioner should ascertain who is available to provide satisfying mutual interpersonal and sexual relationships. The examiner should ask questions of women regarding past pregnancies and deliveries. Women with multiple vaginal deliveries are more likely to have urinary problems while nulliporus women are at a greater risk for breast cancer.

A full description of activity and sleep patterns in a usual 24-hour period, and whether there are recent changes, is an important aspect of the history. If activity or life space is restricted, it should be ascertained whether it is due to fears of urinary dribbling or incontinence. When discussing sleep patterns, the practitioner should determine if sleep is interrupted because of the need to go to the bathroom.

Questions that elicit the ages and reasons for death of parents, grandparents, and siblings are essential aspects of the history. Many diseases of the breast, genital, and urinary systems, such as cancer and diabetes, are genetically linked. The information can help to focus the examiner on a range of potential client problems.

## Past Health History

Previous illnesses or surgery of the breasts, genital, and urinary systems need to be documented and followed-up. For example, if the client had a mastectomy for carcinoma 3 years previous, the practitioner needs to be aware of the possibility of recurrence or metastases. Furthermore, the practitioner should determine the pattern of usual health practices such as the regularity of Papanicolaou (Pap) tests, breast self-examination, and mammography.

## Breasts

The female client may report symmetrical changes in breast contour because of loss of subcutaneous tissue and decreased elasticity of tissues. It is particularly important to obtain a complete history about the breasts, since breast cancer is the most common form of malignancy in the female between 55 and 74 years of age (Silverberg & Lubera, 1987). The regular practice of breast self-exam (BSE) becomes increasingly important to the client who can identify early changes and abnormalities. The nurse must consider if upper extremity mobility and the tactile sense in the finger tips are sufficient to accurately feel the breast before teaching BSE techniques to the older client. An annual mammography is recommended for women over 65. Male clients may report gynecomastia (breast enlargement).

## Urinary System

When present, urinary incontinence is an embarrassing problem for the older individual. It is thought that some form of incontinence is present in approximately 30% of the elderly population (Herzog, Diokno, & Fultz, 1989, p. 83). The incontinent older adult may not readily share information about the problem. Incontinence may be a reason the older adult does not go out of the house. Occasionally, clothing will have a strong urine smell. Because of decreased olfactory sensation, the client may be unaware of the odor. The practitioner needs to ask questions that may indicate the presence and underlying cause of incontinence.

The etiology can include multiple factors such as: decreased mobility, confusion, leakage of urine secondary to stress incontinence, inability to get to the bathroom fast enough, neurologic and cardiovascular disease, diabetes, urinary tract infection, decreased bladder size, or loss of sensation indicating need for micturition. Involuntary bladder contractions are common with the elderly and may be a leading factor in incontinence (Leach & Yip, 1986). Medications such as diuretics or sedatives often contribute to urinary incontinence. If the client is disoriented, the meaning of the urge to void may be confused.

The practitioner needs to carefully ascertain the pattern of the incontinence. The person who is unable to sense the need to void may not be aware of urinating until his or her clothes are wet (reflex or overflow incontinence). The person who is able to sense the need to void, but is unable to delay or control micturition, may urinate on the way to the bathroom (urge incontinence). Stress incontinence may be preceded by a cough or sneeze (Herzog et al., 1989, p. 75). A diary to determine the voiding pattern might prove helpful (Wyman & Fantl, 1988).

A particular problem of the older male is overflow incontinence secondary to prostatic disease or loss of trigone muscle control following prostatic surgery. Dribbling after urinating may be a sign of overflow incontinence secondary to prostatic disease. Females with cystoceles or relaxed musculature from multiple deliveries have an increased incidence of stress incontinence.

Nocturia is frequently reported by the elderly. It occurs with particular frequency in males over 55 years of age who have prostatic enlargement. The practitioner needs to assess whether the client is awakened in response to the urge to void, which may indicate a primary problem relating to the nocturia, or whether the person awakens and just decides to go to the bathroom, which usually indicates a primary problem in sleep pattern. Nocturia is also a common complaint in clients with congestive heart failure due to the increased venous return and kidney perfusion that occur when the client is recumbent.

The kidneys diminish in effectiveness with advancing age, but there should be no renal signs or symptoms in the absence of disease. The older individual is at higher risk of renal insufficiency when increased demands for renal function occur with problems such as dehydration, infection, or congestive heart failure.

## Sexual History

An often omitted area of the history is the sexual history. This may be a function of the discomfort of the practitioner rather than the reluctance of the client to discuss the topic. Although it may be difficult to broach questions regarding sexuality, it is an important aspect of the older person's life.

As for any other age group, the nurse should approach this area with sensitivity to the client's cultural and religious background and life history. By asking questions in a factual but gentle way, the practitioner can help to allay some of the client's anxiety. No special preface, such as, "I am now going to ask some personal questions," is advised, since this only reinforces the client's uneasiness.

In the absence of disease, the capacity of both males and females for sexual intercourse remains present throughout life. Older people often relate positive feelings about their sexual experiences. In the review of systems, the practitioner needs to determine the client's perception of his or her sexual experience, such as satisfaction, availability of partners, discomfort, or self-perception of declining virility or femininity. An open discussion of sexual activity, actual or desired, can reveal areas of concern that are of great significance to the client. Masters and Johnson found that orgasmic experience in older age was directly proportional to frequency of intercourse and orgasm at an earlier age. The older client who was not sexually active at age 45 will probably not be active at age 75 and vice versa (Masters & Johnson, 1966).

The physiologic response to sexual intercourse does change with age. For the male erection occurs more slowly, ejaculation may be of lesser intensity, the volume of seminal fluid may be lessened, and detumescence is more rapid. For the female there is a lessening of muscle tension, diminished vasocongestion (sexual blush), a longer time necessary for lubrication, diminished lubrication, and a lessening in length and intensity of the orgasm.

## Male and Female Genitalia

The main changes in the male genitalia concern the prostate. Prostate problems are so common with advancing age that many men will be aware of the symptoms. A careful history of urination and the outcome of earlier urinary tract examination is appropriate. Men often have misconceptions about prostatic disease, its treatment, and consequences. Here is a time for the practitioner to dispel inaccurate understandings.

A complete childbearing history of the female is essential, since the information may be pertinent to the older female client's gynecologic and urologic problems. The practitioner should obtain a complete history of female menopause including age of onset, symptoms experienced during the transition period, and a history of estrogen replacement therapy, including type and when estrogens were first started. It is also important to determine if the client has experienced any vaginal bleeding or unusual discharge. Any vaginal bleeding occurring one year or more after menopause is considered abnormal and must be referred for follow-up.

## PHYSICAL EXAMINATION

### Breasts

The breasts of both males and females should be examined. Because of testosterone deficiency, male breast enlargement (gynecomastia) may normally occur in older males (see Figure 9.1).

The breasts of the older woman may be pendulous and hang lower because of the forward thrust secondary to kyphosis and the loss of breast and supportive tissues. Special care is needed to examine pendulous breasts. When observing symmetry of the breasts, it is help-

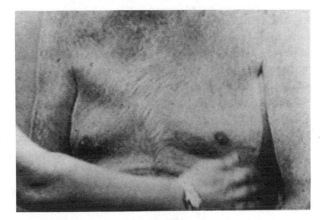

**FIGURE 9.1 Gynecomastia seen in an older man.**

Reprinted with permission from videotape "Physical Assessment of the Aged Person," produced by Herbert H. Lehman College, Department of Nursing, in association with Blue Hill Educational Systems, Inc., under sponsorship of the Research Foundation of the City University of New York, 1975.

ful to ask the client to sit down and lean forward so that the breasts hang away from the chest wall to allow better observation. When palpating the pendulous breast, one hand should be placed on top and one hand beneath the breast so that the simultaneous pressure from the front and back will allow palpation of masses in the pendulous portion. The skin under the breast should be inspected since this area easily can become macerated from perspiration.

Normally no masses will be palpated in the breasts of the older client. The breasts tend to lose their fullness with age because of fibroglandular tissue loss. This loss of breast fullness may make the terminal ducts feel more prominent. These linear, spoke-like strands need to be differentiated from tumor masses. Any palpated mass should be referred for follow-up.

While normally no material can be expressed from the nipples, the nipples may retract secondary to loss in musculature. The differentiating feature of nipple retraction due to aging versus nipple retraction occurring with cancer is that the nipple retracted due to age changes can easily be averted with gentle pressure, and no mass is palpated.

The complete examination of the breasts may be difficult if the older client's movements are severely hampered by arthritis. The practitioner must then make modifications in technique, such as not having the client raise her arms completely over her head. Recumbent positioning, with the arm raised over the head, may also be difficult if the client has a cardiac or respiratory problem. In this case the lowest Fowler's position that can be tolerated should be used.

## Urologic Examination

The skin in the genital area should be observed for redness in the person who has persistent incontinence. Every effort should be made to evaluate incontinence patterns. In individuals with documented or suspected incontinence, stress incontinence can be evaluated while the individual is sitting upright with a pad placed on the perenium. The client is asked to cough several times and the pad is examined for urine. Overflow incontinence may be evaluated by palpating and percussing the bladder following micturation. The palpable bladder would indicate presence of residual urine. The kidneys decrease in size and may be more palpable because the abdominal musculature is decreased.

## Male Genitalia

The male has a lessening and graying of the pubic hair. The perineum becomes less full because of the loss of subcutaneous fat. The penis and testes decrease in size. The testes hang lower and the rugae are diminished in the scrotum because of the loss of muscular tone.

Examination of the prostate is mandatory in the older male as prostatic enlargement increases with age after 40 and is seen in approximately 90% of males by the age of 80 (Berry, 1984). Because of the high incidence of prostatic cancer in males over 75 years of age, it is important to consider the possibility of prostatic cancer when palpating the prostate. Measurement of serum prostate-specific antigen (PSA) may be a helpful addition to rectal examination in early detection of prostate cancer (Catalina, et al. 1991). Prostatic cancer is nearly twice as common in Afro-American males than in whites (Silverberg & Halleb, 1975). Table 9.1 compares physical findings characteristic of benign prostatic hypertrophy (BPH) and cancer of the prostate.

## Female Genitalia

The gynecologic exam should never be overlooked or omitted because of the positive benefit of case finding from both the examination and Pap smear. It is not uncommon for women in the cohort group of 65 and over to exhibit embarrassment while having the examination and to try to talk the practitioner out of performing the examination. During the gynecologic examination, the older woman may find the lithotomy position particularly uncomfortable because of arthritic changes, and a semilithotomy position may be necessary. If the woman has cardiac or respiratory problems, elevation of the head to a semi-Fowler's position may facilitate breathing. When observing the genitalia of an older woman, the nurse will note sparse, britte, and gray pubic hair. The vulva and labia may be smaller because of a loss of subcutaneous fat and decreased estrogen levels. The labia minora, clitoris, and prepuce are usually reduced in size. The skin is usually thin, inelastic, and shiny due to atrophic changes.

The vaginal opening may be narrowed and it may be necessary to use a smaller speculum. It is helpful to insert a finger to check for size of the introitus. The insertion of the speculum is carried out in the usual

**Table 9.1 Physical Findings Characteristic of Benign Prostatic Hypertrophy (BPH) and Cancer of the Prostate**

| Characteristic | BPH | Cancer |
| --- | --- | --- |
| Consistency | Firm | Rock hard |
| Surface | Smooth | Often nodular |
| Symmetry | Symmetrically enlarged | Asymmetrically enlarged |

manner. In the post-menopausal virgin, tightness of the hymen may prevent passage of the speculum.

When inspecting the vagina, the examiner will find a pale thin-appearing vaginal wall. There will be fewer rugae and the atrophic vaginal tissue may bleed easily from the trauma of the speculum insertion. The cervix may be narrowed, shrunken, and appear to be thick and glistening because of estrogen deficiency. With bimanual palpation, a shortened vagina may be felt. The uterus and ovaries may have atrophied and may feel reduced in size.

All older women should be examined closely for signs of cystocele, rectocele, and uterine prolapse, as these are common sequalae of relaxed pelvic musculature. To test for these findings the female client is asked to bear down as though she were going to have a bowel movement and the practitioner observes the vaginal opening. If the vaginal orifice widens or protusion appears, a cystocele, rectocele, or uterine prolapse may be present. The woman is asked to repeat the bearing down while the examiner's finger is in the vagina. With a cystocele, pressure is felt on the anterior surface of the vagina; with a uterine prolapse, protrusion of the cervix is felt down through the vagina.

## NURSING IMPLICATIONS

As with all organ systems, a complete data base will point up client problems or concerns that will allow a wide range of nursing actions (U.S. Department of Health and Human Services, 1991). Early detection of breast and prostate cancer and prevention and early detection of urinary incontinence are major new objectives of health promotion and disease prevention in the elderly. Breast cancer, for example, all too often goes untreated despite the fact that older people have excellent response to treatment. Careful assessment can help the nurse to focus on issues such as breast self-examination, routine mammography, and screening tests for early detection of prostate cancer.

A careful history often suggests simple strategies for reducing symptoms of urinary incontinence in the elderly. For example, if the cause of urinary incontinence is functional because the individual cannot get to the bathroom quickly enough, a portable commode can be placed in the room with the older person which will allow more rapid access to toilet facilities (Newman, Lynch, Smith et al., 1991). Similarly, a simple rescheduling of a diuretic may permit the individual to have a complete night's rest. If constipation is a contributing factor to urinary incontinence, and the client's diet is low in bulk foods, a simple remedy, such as the addition of 2 tablespoons of raw bran to the daily intake, might alleviate the problem (Burton, Pearce, Burgio et al., 1988). On the other hand, symptoms of urinary incontinence may warrant further assessment in order to determine a specific diagnosis. The nurse may choose to perform the additional examination, for example determining a bedside cystometrogram, or to refer the client to an incontinence clinic.

Hydration is important because of the lack of reserve of the older person's kidney function. It should be part of the health maintenance plan to ensure that the older client drinks adequate amounts of fluid daily. During periods of illness, careful observation of intake and output is imperative.

The practitioner should be aware that drugs may affect the elderly differently than they do the young. If the drug is degraded or excreted by the kidneys, the drug concentrations in the elderly may rise to toxic levels because of altered kidney function.

# REFERENCES

Berry, S. J., Coffey D. S., Walsh, P. C., & Ewing L. L. (1984). The development of human benign prostatic hyperplasia with age. The *Journal of Urology, 132,* 474–479.

Burton, J. R., Pearce, L., Burgio, K. L., Engel, B. T., & Whitehead W. E. (1988). Behavioral training for urinary incontinence in elderly ambulatory patients. *Journal of the American Geriatrics Society, 36*,(8) 693–698.

Catalona, W. J. et al. (1991). Measurement of prostate-specific antigen in serum as a screening test for prostate cancer. *New England Journal of Medicine, 324,* 1156.

Herzog, A. R., Diokno, A. C., & Fultz, N. H. (1989). Urinary incontinence: Medical and psychosocial aspects. In Lawton, M. P. (Ed.). *Annual review of gerontology and geriatrics* (p. 83). New York: Springer Publishing Co.

Leach, G. E., & Yip, C. M. (1986). Urologic and urodynamic evaluation of the elderly population. *Clinics in Geriatric Medicine, 2*(4), 731–755.

Masters, W. H., & Johnson, V. E. (1966). *Human sexual response* (pp. 240–241, 262–263). Boston: Little Brown & Co.

Newman, D. K., Lynch, K., Smith, D. A., & Celli, P. (1991). Restoring urinary continence. *American Journal of Nursing, 91*(1), 28–34.

Silverberg, E., & Holleb, A. I. (1975). Major trends in cancer: 25 Year Survey. *A Cancer Journal for Clinicians, 25*(1) 2–8.

Silverberg, E., & Lubera, J. (1987). Cancer statistics, 1987. *A Cancer Journal for Clinicians, 36*(1) 9–25.

U.S. Department of Health and Human Services. (1991). *Healthy people 2000: National health promotion and disease prevention.* Rockville, MD: Public Health Service.

Wyman, J. F., Choi, S. C., Harkins, S. W., Wilson, M. S., & Fantl, J. A. (1988). The urinary diary in evaluation of incontinent women: A test-retest analysis. *Obstetrics and Gynecology*, *71*,(6) 812–817.

# SUGGESTED READINGS

Blair, K. A. (1990). Aging: Physiological aspects and clinical implications. *Nurse Practitioner*, *15*(2), 14–28.

Bretschneider, J. G., & McCoy, N. L. (1988). Sexual interest and behavior in healthy 80- to 102-year-olds. *Archives of Sexual Behavior*, *17*(2), 109–129.

Elipoulous, C. (1990). *Health assessment of the older adult*. (2nd ed.). Redwood City, CA: Addison-Wesley Nursing.

Lierman, L. M., Kasprzyk, D., & Benoliel, J. Q. (1991). Understanding adherence to breast self-examination in older women. *Western Journal of Nursing Research*, *31*(1), 46–66.

McCraken, A. L. (1988). Sexual practice by elders: The forgotten aspect of functional health. *Journal of Gerontological Nursing*, 14(10): 13–18.

Resnick, N. M. (1990). Initial evaluation of the incontinent patient. *Journal of the American Geriatrics Society*, *38*(3), 311–316.

Starr, B. D. (1985). Sexuality and aging. In Eisdorfer, C. (Ed.) *Annual review of gerontology and geriatrics*, Vol. 5. New York: Springer Publishing Co.

Stokes, S. A., Mezey, M. D., & Rauckhorst, L. H. (1975). Respiratory, cardiovascular, breasts, female and male Genitalia. *Physical assessment of the aged person*. (Video tape). Spring Valley, NY: Blue Hill Educational Systems, Inc.

Wyman, J. F. (1988). Nursing assessment of the incontinent geriatric out-patient population. *Nursing Clinics of North America*, *23*(1), 169–187.

# 10

# Musculoskeletal Assessment

## HISTORY

### Client Profile

Gathering information about musculoskeletal functioning begins with an assessment of the client's activity level and functional ability. A thorough discussion of functional assessment can be found in Chapter 4. In addition to functional assessment, the older client should be carefully questioned regarding any perceived changes in musculoskeletal structure and function. The two major disorders of the musculoskeletal system in the elderly are osteoarthritis and osteoporosis. Osteoarthritis, present in 78% of people over 70 years of age, is the most commonly occurring chronic condition of the elderly and can cause marked changes in musculoskeletal functioning and mobility. In postmenopausal women, osteoporosis is associated with 1.3 million fractures annually, of which most are of the vertebrae, wrist, and hip (Prince et al., 1991).

In eliciting the client profile, information about nutrition and exercise is particularly important in developing a profile of people at risk for falls and fractures. Nutritional data should include intake of food products or medications containing calcium, including such over-the-counter medications as "Tums," prior and subsequent to the onset of menopause. The current recommended daily intake of calcium for postmenopausal women is 1,500 milligrams (Consumer Reports, October, 1984). The extent of weight-bearing exercise is important because such exercise can delay or prevent onset of disabilities (Wickham, Walsh, Cooper et al., 1989).

## Past Health History

Past health history related to the musculoskeletal system includes any congenital deformities and past athletic or traumatic injuries, including fractures. A family history of osteoporosis or frequent fractures is pertinent to developing a risk profile for osteoporosis and fractures. A number of medical conditions, including oophorectomy, subtotal gastrectomy, and rheumatoid arthritis can also lead to secondary osteoporosis.

## Review of Systems

The older client should be carefully questioned regarding any perceived changes in musculoskeletal structure and function. Has the client noted any change in muscle bulk, tone, or strength? Has there been any change in the size, shape, or range of motion of joints?

If osteo or rheumatoid arthritis are present or suspected, the practitioner should determine information as to the onset and manifestation of symptoms. Any report of joint or back pain, whether or not previously diagnosed as arthritis, should be fully described as to location, temporal pattern, quality, intensity, and aggravating and relieving factors, because of the high incidence of osteoarthritis. Of special importance is the following information: the degree to which the pain or joint immobility interfere with normal functioning and sleep patterns; current and past use of analgesics, non-steroidals and corticosteroids, including type, dosage, and frequency of administration; and the client's information and attitude toward other medical and to surgical management of the disease. Frequent knee pain associated with osteoarthritis imposes greater limitation on activities such as stair climbing and housekeeping than painless osteoarthritis (Guccione, Felson, & Anderson, 1990).

The client should be questioned as to estrogen replacement therapy, including type, dose, and length of use of estrogen preparations. Information about fluoride and intake of other products for the expressed purpose of preventing osteoporosis should also be obtained. Medications other than calcium and estrogen, which may be relevant to the development of osteoporosis, include thiazide diuretics and sedatives. Long-term use of thiazide diuretics is thought to protect against hip fractures (LaCroix, Weinphal, White et al., 1990). Use of sedatives, especially those with half-lives of greater than 24 hours, is associated with increased risk of hip fracture (Ray, Griffin, Schaffner, Baugh, Melton, 1987). Compression fractures of the vertebrae, often occurring as a consequence of osteoporosis in post-menopausal women, usually present as persistent nonradiating pain in the lumbar spine.

It is not uncommon to elicit a history of muscle cramps occurring in the upper and lower extremities after exercise or at night. While there is often no known physiologic cause for these symptoms, it is important to differentiate the pain from symptoms of intermittent claudication and arteriosclerosis obliterans.

## Falls Risk Assessment

Falls are events that lead to the conscious subject coming to rest inadvertently on the ground (Hindmarsh & Estes, 1989). Only 6% to 10% of falls result in injury, and fewer than 1% result in serious injuries. Nevertheless, falls are the leading cause of accidental death in persons 65 and over, accounting for 33% of the death total (Hindmarsh & Estes, 1989). In addition to injuries, as many as 20% of people who fall say they avoid activities because of a fear of a subsequent fall (Tinetti & Gintner, 1988).

Falls usually occur as a result of the interaction of many factors (Hogue, 1982). A falls "risk profile" (see Table 10.1) is useful in identifying people at risk for injury or of withdrawing from customary activities subsequent to a fall even if no injury has occurred (Mathius & Nayak, 1986).

Postural instability, especially altered balance and gait and increased sway, is clearly associated with increased risk for falling. Several physiologic changes contribute to alterations in stance, balance, and gait, and thus increase the risk of falling in the elderly. Impaired function of nerve endings in the apophyseal joints of the cervical spine and lower extremities impair proprioception and thus impede positioning of the body in space. To compensate, the feet are positioned wider apart, which may cause steps to become irregular and uneven in length. To

**TABLE 10.1 Personal Risk Factors for Falls**

Older age
History of previous falls
Use of sedatives
Cognitive impairment
Visual and hearing impairments
Lower extremity disability and foot problems
Balance and gait abnormalities

maintain balance, the body tends to be bent forward and the hands outstretched (Caranasos & Israel, 1991). As a result, older people, especially women, experience increased sway. Good vision can help compensate for proprioceptive deficits, but when the eyes are closed or vision is diminished, balance is lost. Vestibular dysfunction, common in the elderly, impairs the ability to focus on a moving object while stationary (Caranasos & Israel, 1991). By age 60 to 80, people experience a 20% to 40% decrease in isometric strength; fallers may have an even greater reduction in lower-extremity muscle strength (Hindmarsh & Estes, 1989).

People in their seventies and eighties are more likely to have a shuffling gait characterized by smaller steps, minimal lifting of the feet, and increased time on both feet (see Figure 10.1). Impaired agility makes it harder for people to stand for long periods of time, or to stand on one leg. Symptoms such as light-headedness, dizziness, trouble walking, or past falls should trigger additional questions about gait and balance. When there is no identifiable cause, such complaints of dizziness, unsteadiness, or light-headedness experienced only while walking have been termed benign disequilibrium of aging. This condition can usually be improved by the use of supportive devices (Caranasos & Israel, 1991). Questions that can easily be asked to ascertain gait and balance are shown in Table 10.2.

In addition to gait and balance disturbances, personal risk factors for falls include advanced age, a history of sedative use, prior multiple falls, cognitive impairment, disability of the lower extremities, foot problems, and visual and hearing impairments (Tinetti, Speechley, &

---

**TABLE 10.2 Questions to Ascertain Balance and Gait**

Do you have any difficulty rising from a chair? Do you use both arms? If so, do you use them evenly?
Do you feel unstable when you walk? Stand? Rise from a chair?
Have you noticed any muscle weakness in your legs?
Have you noticed any change in your stride length or walking speed?
Do you find that you are unsteady when walking on soft surfaces?
Are you hesitant when walking?
Do you swing both arms evenly when walking?

---

*Notes.* From "Gait Assessment in the Elderly: A Gait Abnormality Rating Scale and its Relation to Falls," by L. Wolfson, R. Whipple, P. Amerman, and J. Tobin, 1990, *Journals of Gerontology, 45,* pp. M12–19.

From "Risk Factors for Recurrent Nonsyncopal Falls," by M. Nevitt, S. Cummings, S. Kidd, and D. Black, 1989, *Journal of the American Medical Association, 261,* pp. 2663–2668.

From "Effects of Walking on Balance Among Elders," by B. Roberts, 1989, *Nursing Research, 38,* pp. 180–182.

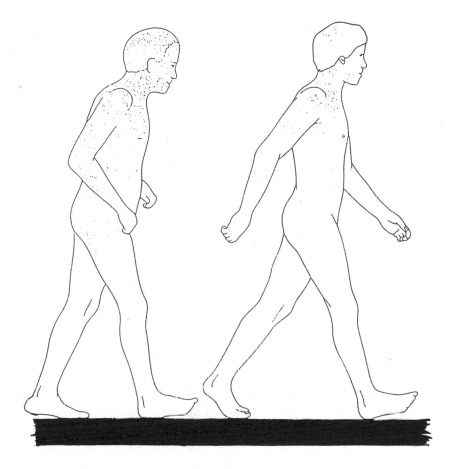

**FIGURE 10.1 Characteristic gait of the elderly as contrasted to younger people.**

Reproduced with permission. Caranasos, G. & Israel, R. (1991). "Gait Disorders in the Elderly." *Hospital Practice*, *26*(6), 75. Illustration by Laura Pardi Duprey.

Ginter, 1988). Having several of these risk factors greatly enhances the risk of falling. Multiple stumbles within the past month have also been associated with an increased risk of falling (Teno, Keil, & Mor, 1990).

Tripping over loose objects on the floor and inadequately lit or marked stair treads are the most frequently cited environmental hazards contributing to falls. Also implicated are clothes lying on the floor, loose carpet edges and unanchored throw rugs, and loose tiles in bathrooms and kitchens.

## PHYSICAL EXAMINATION

## Upper Extremities

In examining the hands, muscle bulk may be diminished symmetrically in association with wasting of fine muscles. Manifestations of chronic illnesses may be evident. Heberden's nodes, enlargement or change in the configuration of the distal, interphalangeal joints of the fingers are indicative of osteoarthritis (see Figure 10.2). These lesions are nonpainful and usually do not result in deficits in function. Dupuytren's contractures, on the other hand, present as an overgrowth and contraction of palmar fascia, which involves the ring and other fingers, and do progressively impair function of the hand. Dupuytren's contractures occur more often in older Caucasian men and increase in frequency with age (see Figure 10.3). The practitioner should note evidence of any involuntary movements of the upper extremities, which may be indicative of senile tremors or the tremors of Parkinson's disease. If the client has rheumatoid arthritis, the typical deformities should be noted.

In the upper extremities, muscle tone, elicited by palpation of a muscle while putting a joint through passive range of motion, is often diminished symmetrically. The degree of muscle strength should correlate with muscle bulk. The strength of the hand grip is usually well preserved. The client can usually adequately perform range of motion of the joints of the upper extremities. However, the practitioner can expect to find some evidence of joint stiffness and crepitation with advanced age. When present, crepitation is felt as a grating sensation when a joint is palpated throughout range of motion.

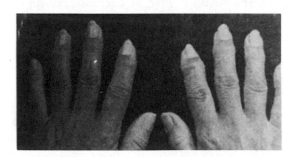

**FIGURE 10.2 Heberden's Nodes commonly seen with osteoarthritis.**

From Hollander, J. L. & McCarty, D. J. 1972. *Arthritis and Allied Conditions*, 8th Ed. Philadelphia: Lea and Febiger. Reproduced with permission.

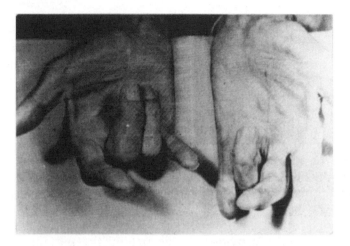

**FIGURE 10.3 Dupuytren's contracture of both hands.**

From McDowell, F. 1971. Plastic Surgery. In Cowdry, E.V. & Steinberg, F.U. (Eds.) The *Care of the Geriatric Patient*, 4th Ed. St. Louis: C.V. Mosby Co. Reproduced with permission.

## Lower Extremities

The findings related to muscle mass, bulk, and strength are similar to those found in the upper extremities. Examination includes assessment of the full range of motion and muscle strength of all major muscle groups, especially the hips and knees. Straight leg-raising should be performed to check for the possibility of spinal stenosis. Fasciculations, or involuntary movements, are commonly seen in the calf muscles of older men. (For vascular examination of the lower extremities, see Chapter 7).

Osteoarthritis is especially evident in the weight-bearing joints of the lower extremities (Kane, Ouslander, & Abrams, 1989). If present, there will be synovial thickening and crepitation, with a concomitant decrease in range of motion and/or pain on motion or weight-bearing. (A discussion of feet and nails is found in Chapter 5).

## Gait and Balance

Assessment of gait and balance involves three elements: posture, standing balance, and gait. Posture is assessed by observing the client walk, sit, and stand during the course of the encounter. Although many tests of balance and gait are impractical for use in the clinical setting, certain tests and maneuvers are easily adapted and are recommended for inclusion in the physical examination of all older adults. If time or resources do not permit assessment of every client, assessment can be reserved for people at risk; for example, clients reporting falls and injuries and those with diseases that make them more likely to fall, such as severe arthritis or Parkinson's disease.

Balance can be assessed by having the client stand with legs apart and then together with eyes open and then closed. The Romberg test is more fully discussed in Chapter 12. Sway, which generally increases with aging, may increase even more in the absence of visual cues (Caranasos & Israel, 1991).

The nudge test is used to check for backwards falling. To perform the nudge test, the provider stands behind the patient, with arms looped around the patient, and gently presses on the sternum. Most older people can sustain a nudge without losing their balance. Easy displacement backward is seen in Parkinson's disease, cervical spondylosis, and normal pressure hydrocephalus (Hindmarsh & Estes, 1989; Caranasos & Israel, 1991).

The "get up and go" test provides a useful measure of balance and gait in the elderly (Mathius & Nayak, 1986; Podsiadlo & Richardson, 1991). While seated in an armless, straight-backed chair, the client is asked to rise without using the arms of the chair to help them stand up, stand still briefly, walk forward 10 feet toward a wall, turn around without touching the wall, walk back to the chair, turn around and sit down. The client can be offered a trial run before the actual test. Two measures for scoring are reported. The original scoring has no time limitation; the observer rates the client on a 5-point scale with 1 normal and 5 severely abnormal. Intermediate scores are assigned based on speed, hesitancy, abnormal movement of the trunk or upper limbs, staggering, and stumbling (Podsiadlo & Richardson, 1991). The time needed in seconds to complete the task has been suggested as an alternate scoring method (Evans & Rosenberg, 1991). Elderly clients without impairment can complete the test within 10 seconds or less. People who take more than 30 seconds to complete the test tend to be dependent in ability to shower, get in and out of bed, or climb stairs.

Fall rating scales, such as those developed by Tinetti, also provide valid and reliable information about a person's balance and gait (Tinetti & Gintner, 1988; Mathius & Nayak, 1986). Items are scored depending on the person's ability to sit, balance, rise from a sitting position, ability to stand with eyes open and closed, and turning balance. The nudge test is also often included in the battery of maneuvers. Gait maneuvers in many falls assessment instruments include initiation of gait, step height and symmetry, and walking stance. Many scales have specific directions as to how they should be administered.

As with all areas of functional assessment, no tests performed in the office substitute for observation of the client's balance and gait in his or her own home. Evaluation of mobility in the client's own space can help ascertain, for example, how the placement of furniture assists or impedes mobility. Similarly, a home visit is especially useful in determining the effective use of assistive devices; for example, raised toilet seats, the client's ability to move up and down stairs, and the nature of barriers to entering or leaving the home. Such an evaluation, ideally performed in conjunction with an occupational or physical therapist, can add immeasurably to the understanding and improvement of mobility problems.

## IMPLICATIONS FOR PRACTICE

A plan for promoting postural alignment and a balance of activity and rest is an important part of the health maintenance plan for every older client. This is necessary not only to maintain muscle strength and joint range of motion, but also to enhance body image and sense of well-being. Exercise can also improve physiologic parameters such as respiratory status. Prevention of excessive weight gain is especially important, for example in the management of arthritis, since extra weight puts additional stress on damaged weight-bearing joints (see Chapter 8 for a more complete discussion of weight and nutrition).

An exercise program should include activity for both large and small muscle groups through stretching and reaching-out exercises and adequate range of motion of major joints. Exercises to improve flexibility, fitness, and endurance substantially improve musculoskeletal status, cardiovascular function, and metabolic markers of aging, even for people in their late seventies and eighties who have led sedentary lifestyles (Evans & Rosenberg, 1991). It may be helpful to refer the client to special exercise classes sponsored by health agencies or community groups.

Safety is a major concern of older people. Safety considerations related to self-administration of medications such as analgesics for arthritic pain include monitoring the client's pattern of drug taking (frequency and dosage) as well as observing for side effects. Teaching should be directed toward promotion of self-care activities that achieve optimum therapeutic effect with a minimum safety hazard.

Prevention of fractures and other injuries is of special concern and a major focus of health prevention activities for the elderly (U.S. Department of Health and Human Services, 1991). There is now substantial evidence that estrogen replacement therapy, along with calcium intake and exercise, lessens the risk of fractures in the elderly (Prince, Smith, Dick et al., 1991). Estrogen replacement requires careful administration and monitoring for endometrial and breast cancer. Adequate maintenance of calcium requires intake of 1,500 mg/24 hours. To achieve these levels, many people use calcium supplements as they are unable to take in sufficient calcium in their daily diet (for example, 5 to 6 cups of milk).

Information about the older client's living arrangements may indicate a need to eliminate common causes of falls. Environmental hazards and certain medications are particularly implicated as contributing to more falls. Stairs should be well lit, have hand rails on both sides, and rises which are marked with contrasting colors. Nonskid tub mats and wall bars in the bathroom may provide added safety. This is especially important for the older client who has a visual deficit, unsteady balance, or a shuffling gait. Medications which have been implicated as contributing to falls, for example, long-acting benzodiazipins, should be avoided when at all possible. Referral to a falls assessment and prevention program may be appropriate.

# REFERENCES

Caranasos, G., & Israel R. (1991). Gait disorders in the elderly. *Hospital Practice*.

*Consumer Reports*. Osteoporosis. October, 1984. pp. 576–580.

Evans, W., & Rosenberg, I.H. (1991). *Biomarkers: The 10 determinants of aging you can control*. New York: Simon & Shuster.

Guccione, A., Felson, D., & Anderson, J. (1990). Defining arthritis and measuring functional status in elders: Methodological issues in the study of disease and physical disability. *American Journal of Public Health, 80*, 945–949.

Handmarsh, J., & Estes, H. (1989). Falls in older persons: Causes and interventions. *Archives of Internal Medicine, 149*, 2217–2222.

Hogue, C. (1982). Injury in late life, I: Epidemiology. *Journal of the American Geriatric Society, 30*, 183–190.

Kane, R., Ouslander, J., & Abrass, I. (1989). *Essentials of clinical geriatrics*. New York: McGraw Hill Information Services Co.

LaCroix, A., Wienpahl, J., White, L., et al. (1990). Thiazide diuretic agents and the incidence of hip fracture. *New England Journal of Medicine, 322*, 286–290.

Mathius, S., Nayak, U. L., & Isaacs, B. (1986). Balance in elderly patients: The "Get Up and Go" test. *Archives of Physical Medicine and Rehabilitation, 67*, 387–389.

Podsiadlo, D., & Richardson, S. (1991). The timed "up & go": A test of basic functional mobility for frail elderly persons. *Journal of the American Geriatric Society, 39*, 142–147.

Prince, R., Smith, M., Dick, I. et al. (1991). Prevention of postmenopausal osteoporosis: A comparative study of exercise, calcium supplementation, and hormone-replacement therapy. *New England Journal of Medicine, 325,* 1189–1195.

Ray, W., Griffin, M., Schaffner, W., Baugh, K., & Melton, L. (1987). Psychotropic drug use and the risk of hip fracture. *New England Journal of Medicine, 316,* 363–369.

Teno, J., Keil, D., & Mor, V. (1990). Multiple stumbles: A risk factor for falls in community-dwelling elderly. *Journal of the American Geriatrics Society, 38,* 1321–1325.

Tinetti, M. E., & Gintner S. (1988). Identifying mobility dysfunctions in elderly patients: Standard neuromuscular examination or direct assessment? *Journal of the American Medical Association, 259,* 1190–1193.

Tinetti, M. E., Speechley, M., & Ginter, S. (1988). Risk factors for falls among elderly persons living in the community. *New England Journal of Medicine, 319,* 1701–1707.

U.S. Department of Health and Human Services. (1991). *Healthy people 2000: Health promotion and disease prevention.* Rockville, MD: Public Health Service.

Wickham, C., Walsh, K., Cooper, C. et al. (1989). Dietary calcium, physical activity and risk of hip fracture: A prospective study. *British Medical Journal, 299,* 889–892.

## SUGGESTED READINGS

Burke, M., & Walsh, M. (1992). *Gerontological nursing: Care of the frail elderly.* St. Louis: Mosby YearBook Inc.

Chenitz, W. C., Stone, J., & Salisbury, S. (1991). *Clinical gerontological nursing: A guide to advanced practice* (Chapters 5 & 14). Philadelphia: W.B. Saunders Co.

Eliopoulos, C. (1990). *Health Assessment of the Older Adult.* Redwood City, CA: Addison-Wesley Nursing, A Division of the Benjamin/Cummings Publishing Co., Inc.

Lavizzo-Mourey, R., Day, S., Diserens, D., & Grisso, J. (1989). *Practicing prevention for the elderly* (Chapters 9 and 10). Philadelphia: Hanley & Belfus Inc.

Lord, S., Clark, R., & Webster, I. (1991). Postural stability and associated physiological factors in a population of aged persons. *Journals of Gerontology, 46,* M69-76.

Luechenotte, A. (1990). *Pocket guide to gerontologic assessment.* St. Louis: Mosby YearBook, Inc.

MacDonald, J. (1985). Falls in the elderly: The role of drugs in the elderly. *Clinical Geriatric Medicine, 1,* 621–636.

# 11

# Assessment of Mental/Emotional Status

Older people worry about their mental health. In particular, they are concerned that loss of memory may negatively affect their day-to-day ability to care for themselves and to function independently, for example, to continue to drive a car. There is also wide concern that changes in mental functioning may herald the onset of dementia. Older people who are admitted to a hospital worry about becoming confused and needing to be restrained. In long-term care facilities, decline in mental functioning often results in relocation to a more structured and, from the resident's viewpoint, less desirable unit within the facility.

Despite, or perhaps because of these concerns, many older people are reluctant to share perceived changes in mental status with a health care professional. Rather, they present to the primary caregiver with vague physical symptoms or disturbances in functioning, such as inability to sleep. Symptoms of depression may go unmentioned or be mistaken for normal age changes. Some older people and their families, on the other hand, seek an encounter with a health professional for the expressed purpose of a complete assessment of mental functioning. Such patients may present with grave concerns about symptoms of memory changes or unexplained or inappropriate mood swings or behavior changes. A thorough history and mental/emotional status examination may be sufficient to reassure people that their symptoms are consistent with the normal aging process.

Nevertheless, as they age, people have reason to be concerned about their mental health. All together, more than 18% of older people are thought to evidence significant mental health problems at any given time, and the incidence of altered mental functioning increases substantially in older age (Gottleib, 1989). Some older people have long-standing mental health disabilities which may be exacerbated as they age. Others manifest new mental and emotional problems related to changes in social or physical functioning, for example, situational depressions associated with loss of social supports and increasing frailty. Still others, especially the very old, are at risk for developing dementia. The two most commonly diagnosed true dementias are Alzheimer's Disease (AD), which accounts for 50% to 70% of all dementias, and Multi Infarct Dementia (MID).

Thus, identification of early symptoms of mental/emotional disorders is important in that it can trigger a more complete work-up, treatment, and early referral to appropriate resources.

## HISTORY

Assessment of mental/emotional status occurs simultaneously both during history-taking and as part of the physical examination. During the interview the practitioner hears the client's verbal responses, observes nonverbal behavior, and elicits subjective data concerning the client's self-perception and ability to function in the environment. The physical examination provides objective evidence of cognition and affect. The most complete picture of a person's mental functioning comes from a blending of the history and physical examination data.

## Client Profile

Judgments about a person's mental/emotional status begin immediately on encountering the client. By listening to and observing people's responses to questions, the nurse determines fluidity of thought and expression, ability to concentrate, correctness, appropriateness and consistency, and the richness and detail of information provided by the patient. Animation about or avoidance of topics alerts the practitioner to potential areas of stress or conflict.

For people who are reluctant to reveal symptoms that may indicate decline in mental capacity, careful, systematic, and sympathetic questioning can help to identify the true reason for a visit. Older people who recognize that they are experiencing memory changes may attempt to mask such changes. Confabulation or vague responses to objective questions can alert the interviewer to such behaviors, which may be early signs of dementia. In contrast, dwelling on symptoms and communicating a strong sense of distress may be signs of depression.

Attempts should be made to elicit data descriptive of the client's self-concept and how the person feels about his or her life situation. It is important to ascertain information about the client's personality and coping styles in earlier life, as patterns tend to persist over the life cycle. The practitioner needs to determine whether the client's current perceptions and behavior are congruent with previous patterns before judging them to be age-related changes.

The family is often a good source of information about the general demeanor and personality of the older person. Has the person been a lifelong risk-taker or has she or he been risk averse? Does the person rise to a challenge through careful consideration of options, immediate action, or withdrawal? What role does the older person play within her or his circle of family and friends?

## Past Health History

As at any age, a past history of psychiatric symptoms and treatment, as well as central nervous system trauma or surgery, is relevant. The history includes data concerning drugs that the client has taken in the past or is presently taking. Examples of pertinent medications include: central nervous system stimulants or depressants; tranquilizers, mood elevators, and other drugs that may alter mood and affect (for example, corticosteroids and anticholinergics); sedatives; and substances such as alcohol or drugs that alter central nervous system functioning.

## Family History

Eliciting a family history of alcoholism, depression, abuse, and/or dementia can provide a framework for a preventive approach. The practitioner can anticipate questions and concerns of elderly patients. For example, patients with a family history of dementia will have concerns about the familial nature of the disease.

The family history also provides an opportunity to assess social functioning and the availability of social supports. Social supports play a major role in both preventing mental/emotional illness, and in assisting people with and without mental health problems to remain in the community. Various aspects of social functioning that are important to assess in the elderly include coping and subjective sense of well-being, feelings of being loved and cared about, feelings that help is available, availability of social contacts, and environmental resources (Newman, Struyk, Wright, & Rice, 1990).

Coping and subjective well-being encompasses such constructs as subjective sense of self, happiness, morale, life satisfaction, future orientation, and skill and sense of mastery over the environment. Questions to ascertain subjective well-being can be as simple as, "How would you rate your health at the present time?" "Would you call yourself old, middle-aged, or young? Do you have many, few, no, plans for next year? Most practitioners find these simple, one item questions sufficient for primary care practice.

The practitioner will want a detailed picture of an older person's social interactions and social and environmental resources. Such data include the number and type of people with whom the older person interacts, often referred to as the density and diversity of the person's social network. Of prime importance are the nature, quality, and reciprocity of social interactions, available social resources should the client become ill, and environmental resources and constraints both within the home (bathing and cooking facilities, for example) and in the community (for example, accessibility to shopping, health providers and facilities, and transportation).

Although much of the social history is collected throughout the health encounter, quantifiable instruments may prove helpful in expanding the practitioner's repertoire of questions, and might also be incorporated into the health assessment. The Family APGAR, (Table 11.1), for example, yields information about an older person's satisfaction with family relationships and supports (Kane & Kane, 1988). Other instruments provide explicit information about contacts with children, other family, and friends, along with a general measure of satisfaction with resources. (Kane & Kane, 1988). Such instruments are easy to administer, can be completed by the client alone or by the client and provider together, and can serve as a point of departure for further exploration of social supports.

## Review of Systems

The review of systems allows for precise and systematic clarification as to the client's current mental/emotional status. The practitioner should ascertain any changes of concern to the client. If the client acknowledges any strong preoccupations or altered thought processes, such as fears, phobias, hypochondriasis, or feelings of worthlessness, it is important to ascertain the extent to which they interfere with daily functioning.

As at any age, high levels of stress can exacerbate mental/emotional or organic illness. Advancing age can be associated with a number of stresses, such as loss of loved ones, functional abilities, health, and

## TABLE 11.1 Family APGAR

*Adaptation*
1. I am satisfied with the help that I receive from my family when something is troubling me.

*Partnership*
2. I am satisfied with the way my family discusses items of common interest and shares problem-solving with me.

*Growth*
3. I find that my family accepts my wishes to take on new activities and make changes in my lifestyle.

*Affection*
4. I am satisfied with the way my family expresses affection and responds to my feelings such as anger, sorrow, and love.

*Resolve*
5. I am satisfied with the way my family and I share time together.

Scoring
　　(2) almost always
　　(1) some of the time
　　(0) hardly ever

*Note.* Adapted from "The family APGAR: A proposal for a family function test and its use by physicians" by G. Smilkstein, 1978, *Journal of Family Practice*, *6*, pp. 1231–1239. Copyright © 1978. Reprinted with permission of Appleton & Lange, Inc.

material goods. Often these stresses occur over a compressed period of time. It is important to ascertain the number, time of occurrence, and significance of losses. Family members or friends may provide clarifying data and the practitioner should note how well these data corroborate information obtained from the client. The Gordon/Stokes Stress Scale (Table 11.2) provides an objective measure of the number and severity of life changes. Persons with high life stress scores are at greater risk for developing mental/emotional or physical health problems (Gordon & Stokes, 1988).

Additional portions of the review of systems which may reveal symptoms relevant to assessment of mental/emotional status include, for example, changes in vision, hearing, equilibrium, speech, and bowel and bladder control, as well as aspects of the neurological history such as headaches, seizures, head injuries and changes in level of consciousness.

## PHYSICAL EXAMINATION

### General Appearance and Behavior

General appearance and behavior are noted at the beginning of the interview. Included are the appropriateness of the older person's dress and grooming for age, sex, and climate. It is important to look for fac-

## TABLE 11.2 The Stokes/Gordon Stress Scale (SGSS)

**Directions:** Below are listed events and situations which occur in everyday life. Place an X next to any event or situation you are currently experiencing.

____ 1. Change in your sleeping habits (such as ability to fall or stay asleep, change in place of sleep, etc.)

____ 2. Decreasing number of friends or losing old friends

____ 3. Giving up or losing driver's license

____ 4. Personality characteristics of your husband or wife are more annoying than before

____ 5. Time with children or grandchildren too short

____ 6. Foreclosure of mortgage or loan

____ 7. Change in behavior of family member

____ 8. Taking relative or friend into your home to live

____ 9. Fear of your own or your husband's or wife's driving

____ 10. Change in your responsibilities at work

____ 11. Major change in number of family get togethers

____ 12. Fired from work or being laid off

____ 13. Change in your diet or eating habits

____ 14. Difficulty making new friends

____ 15. Change in residence by moving to a new home

____ 16. Concern for completing required forms (such as income tax, Medicare forms, etc.)

____ 17. Thinking about your own death

____ 18. Slowing down

____ 19. Disturbing dreams

____ 20. Difficulty dealing with children or grandchildren (such as noise, mess, etc.)

____ 21. Minor violation of the law (such as traffic violation, jay-walking, disturbing the peace, etc.)

____ 22. Feeling of remaining time being short

____ 23. Feeling of being taken advantage of by "the system" (such as clinics, Medicare, social security, etc.)

____ 24. Change in social activities (such as clubs, dancing, visiting, entertaining, etc.)

____ 25. Constant or recurring pain or discomfort

____ 26. Change in residence by moving in with children or other family members

____ 27. Change in recreational activities (such as golf, tennis, walking, theatre attendance, etc.)

____ 28. Change in your working hours or conditions

____ 29. Making out a will

____ 30. Holiday (such as Christmas, Rosh Hashanah, 4th of July, etc.)

____ 31. Change to different line of work

____ 32. Being away from home overnight or longer (such as vacation, visits, etc.)

____ 33. Vacation

____ 34. Anniversary

____ 35. Retirement

*(continued)*

**TABLE 11.2** (*continued*)

_____ 36. Reaching a milestone year (becoming 65, 70, 75, 80, 85, 90)
_____ 37. Change in your sexual activity
_____ 38. Dependency on other people
_____ 39. Using your savings for living expenses
_____ 40. Needing to rely on cane, wheelchair, walker, or hearing aid
_____ 41. Loneliness or aloneness
_____ 42. Inability to get out of the house
_____ 43. Minor or major car accident
_____ 44. Illness or injury of husband or wife
_____ 45. Illness or injury of son, daughter, or grandchild
_____ 46. Illness or injury of close relative (such as sister, brother, parent, etc.)
_____ 47. Your own hospitalization (unplanned)
_____ 48. Your own hospitalization (planned)
_____ 49. Hospitalization of husband or wife
_____ 50. Hospitalization of son, daughter, or grandchild
_____ 51. Not having enough money for food or medicine
_____ 52. Illness in public places (such as uncontrollable behavior, wetting, passing out, etc.)
_____ 53. Change in style of living because of lack of money
_____ 54. Fear of being a victim of a street crime
_____ 55. Decreasing mental abilities (such as forgetting, difficulty with decision-making, planning, etc.)
_____ 56. Being judged legally incompetent
_____ 57. Pressure for increased socializing
_____ 58. Son or daughter leaving home
_____ 59. Wife or husband begins or stops work
_____ 60. Uncertainty about the future
_____ 61. Trouble with your boss
_____ 62. Wanting events to go well with people seen infrequently (such as visits, parties, etc.)
_____ 63. Too much closeness or time with husband or wife (result of retirement, etc.)
_____ 64. Outstanding personal achievement
_____ 65. Your remarriage
_____ 66. Addition of a new family member (through birth, marriage, adoption, etc.)
_____ 67. Regret for not having done something you wanted to do in life (such as having children, getting a college education, etc.)
_____ 68. Change in religious activities
_____ 69. Death of a grandchild
_____ 70. Death of a son or daughter (unanticipated or unexpected)
_____ 71. Death of son or daughter (anticipated or expected)
_____ 72. Death of husband or wife (unanticipated or unexpected)
_____ 73. Death of husband or wife (anticipated or expected)
_____ 74. Death of other close family member (such as sister, brother, parent, etc.)
_____ 75. Death of close friend
_____ 76. Death of loved pet
_____ 77. Change in ability to do own personal care (such as bathing, dressing, etc.)

(*continued*)

____ 78. Your own personal injury or illness
____ 79. Change in residence by moving to an institution
____ 80. Concern for children (such as out of work, divorce, arguments, etc.)
____ 81. Inability to care for yourself
____ 82. Decreasing eyesight
____ 83. Loss of ability to get around due to illness or aging
____ 84. Divorce or legally separating from your husband or wife
____ 85. Being separated from husband or wife (such as admission to hospital or nursing home, vacation, etc.)
____ 86. Having an unexpected debt (such as hospital bills, etc.)
____ 87. Concern for grandchildren
____ 88. Decreasing hearing
____ 89. Fear of your home being invaded or robbed
____ 90. Going to jail
____ 91. Son or daughter moving back into house
____ 92. Change in your financial state
____ 93. Taking on a significant debt (such as mortgage, loan, etc.)
____ 94. Not enough visits to or from family members
____ 95. Wishing parts of your life had been different
____ 96. Not feeling needed or having a purpose in life
____ 97. Giving up long-cherished possessions (such as home, dishes, pictures, etc.)
____ 98. Longing for or missing children or grandchildren
____ 99. Fear of abuse from others (such as family, associates, strangers, etc.)
____100. Concern about elimination (such as constipation, diarrhea, difficulty urinating, etc.)
____101. Concern for world conditions
____102. Increase in arguments, bickering, or disagreements with your husband or wife
____103. Reconciliation with your husband or wife
____104. Difficulty using public transportation system

*Note.* From S. Stokes and S. Gordon, 1987. Reprinted with permission.

---

tors indicating demeanor, such as apparent age, posture, position assumed, and facial expressions.

The nurse will also want to note the client's general level of responsiveness to the environment and the client's energy and motor activity level. Where does the client look? Is there eye contact? Is the client aware of environmental stimuli or is he or she very distractible? Is the client inert or restless? What gestures or mannerisms are observable? It is also important to note whether the older client observes the usual expected social amenities that are congruent with sociocultural background. Particular note should be taken of any extremes of behavior during the history taking or physical examination, for example, constant fidgeting, apathy, or hostility.

## Level of Consciousness

In assessing level of consciousness, both the rapidity and correctness of the older client's response to verbal questions should be assessed. Level of consciousness is initially assessed with simple, one-level commands such as: "Touch your nose." An example of a second-level command would be "Wrinkle your nose and touch your ear;" a third-level command: "Take this piece of paper, fold it in half, and place it on the floor." Normally, the older client is alert and should be able to answer questions presented by the practitioner promptly and with accuracy. If the client erroneously answers questions that would ordinarily be answered correctly, the practitioner should check for decreased hearing or vision which may distort findings. Mild decreases in level of consciousness in the older person may be an early sign of an acute illness or neurologic disturbance. Clients with a mild decrease in level of consciousness will tire easily, become inattentive, and/or show a fluctuating level of response to the interviewer. Such a client may not perform as well in response to second- or third-level commands.

## Stream of Mental Activity, Verbal Spontaneity, and Productivity

In the older person, as in other age groups, mental activity, verbal spontaneity, and productivity vary with educational level, life experience, and cultural norms. The older person who has been socially isolated and has had limited stimulation and restricted life experience may be less spontaneous and flexible. Older persons are likely to be spontaneously verbal about topics in which they are interested such as health, transportation, handling of money, or activities of daily living. Therefore, if an older client is responding to questions only in monosyllables, an attempt should be made to ascertain primary areas of concern or interest to the client and to use nondirective techniques to elicit spontaneous verbalizations.

## Thought Content

Themes of special significance to the older person, such as self-image, self-assessment of health, and perceptions of life space and of the outside world, usually become evident during the course of the history. Table 11.3 presents an example of a brief interview to elicit thought content.

Seeing oneself as "old" has a negative connotation in our youth-oriented culture. Despite this, research findings indicate that through-

**TABLE 11.3 Questions to Elicit Thought Content Themes**

| | |
|---|---|
| Introduction | I will be asking you some questions to learn more about you and how you see yourself. |
| Activity pattern | What kinds of things do you do on a typical day? (Elicits data regarding life space, friends, social contacts, spheres of interest.) |
| | Have you noticed any changes in your daily activities of social contacts? |
| | Were you a more active person earlier in life? |
| Self-image | Can you share with me any feelings you have about getting older? |
| | How do you feel about your health now? |
| Life satisfaction | What kinds of things give you the most satisfaction? |
| and concerns | What kinds of things do you worry about? |
| Life changes | What are the major changes that you have experienced as you have grown older? |

out the life span, self-ratings do not appreciably change with aging. Older persons who are unable to see their own worth may be depressed. However, it is characteristic of older people to show increased concern regarding health status and bodily functions. (Refer to Chapter 2, Growth and Development of the Older Person, for further discussion of self-image.)

The richness and diversity of thought content in older persons is related to the range of their current life experiences. Those with frequent new life experiences will show more richness of thought content than those who are socially isolated. Even when mental status is normal, socially isolated older persons may show poverty of thought content regarding current life experiences, and it may be more productive to discuss past life experiences. Anxiety about existing or anticipated health problems may prevent older people from focusing on topics other than their health. Similarly, thought content will be constricted for those older clients whose life space is limited to a narrow geographic area and who see themselves as having a limited range of social roles and obligations.

## Affect, Mood, and Emotional Reactions

The older client should exhibit the normal range of appropriate emotions. As at any age, extremes of emotional display, or displays of emotions that are inappropriate to the situation, require further assessment. Organic brain disease, for example, stroke or dementias, can cause lability of affect. Such variability in mood and emotional reactions may be characterized by sudden unexplained episodes of crying or laughter.

## Language Ability

Vocabulary and the fund of general information normally increase with advancing age. There are no major changes in speech patterns characteristic of normal aging. Therefore, any significant change in expressive language ability requires further investigation.

## Cognition

Cognitive function encompasses orientation, remote and recent memory, perceptual and psychomotor ability, concentration, judgment and abstract reasoning, reaction time, learning ability, and intelligence (Kane & Kane, 1988). Assessing cognition is particularly important in the elderly because cognitive changes may be the first sign of dementia, and because eligibility for long-term care services is often linked to level of cognitive function.

When asking the older client questions to elicit level of orientation to time, place, and person, the practitioner should expect no deterioration or change with normal aging. The client should be able to correctly state the date and time of day, where he or she is, and identify who he or she is, and/or the names of family members. If there is an apparent loss of specific time orientation (for example, the client is unable to state the exact date of the month), the interviewer should determine whether this may be due to social isolation rather than deterioration in mental functioning.

Ability to recall both remote and recent memories is tested extensively during the course of the health history. There is no change in memory associated with normal aging. Immediate recall can be tested by asking the client to repeat a short series of numbers or words (for example, the names of three commonly encountered objects) within a limited time frame. Accurate retention of a series of five digits or three or more common objects by the older client is considered normal.

Speaking with family members can provide invaluable information. For example, family may have noticed an increase in the need to repeat information, changes in ability to keep the house clean, or deterioration in eating mannerisms, and they can provide additional information not otherwise apparent to the practitioner.

In assessing abstract intellectual function, while norms for assessment in older persons provide for a wider range of errors than for young adults, the older person should be able to perform tests that involve memory, concentration, comprehension, and abstraction. Such tests can involve the following techniques: counting and one-step arithmetic calculations (for example, counting by twos); verbal insight by explanation of a proverb (for example, "A stitch in time saves nine"); or analogies (for example, "How are a bus and train alike?). Some deterioration may be noted in verbal insight. For example, the client may be more concrete or less accurate in explaining the meaning of proverbs or analogies. Usually, there is little or no change in these abilities before age 65; a sharper decrease may occur after age 75.

In addition to the traditional history questions, short, easily administered scales of cognitive functioning are the most widely used initial measures of mental status in the elderly. Examples of easily administered measures of cognitive function and one example of a performance test follow.

*The Mini-Mental State Examination (MMS)* (Table 11.4). Perhaps the most commonly used scale for assessing cognitive function in the elderly, the MMS, or "Folstein," has 11 questions which assess both verbal responses and performance (Folstein, Folstein, & McHugh, 1975). With practice the test can easily be administered in 5 to 10 minutes and has been shown to differentiate clearly between patients with delirium, dementia, and depression as opposed to normal controls. The highest (perfect) MMS score is 30. Scores of 21 or below are associated with dementia, delirium, or affective disorders (Folstein et al., 1975). Scores between 21 and 24 have been described by some as constituting a "grey" zone of potential delirium or dementia.

*The Short Portable Mental Status Questionnaire (SPMSQ)* (Table 11.5). The SPMSQ was developed as part of the comprehensive assessment battery of instruments included in the Older Americans Research and Service Center Instrument (OARS) (Pfeiffer, 1975). The spread of possible scores is between 0 and 10. Scores allow for differentiation among 4 levels of disability: 0-2 errors (a score of 8 or higher) indicates intact cognition; more frequent errors differentiate among mild, moderate and severe intellectual impairment. Scoring takes into account educational level and race.

*The Face-Hand Test.* The face-hand test may be particularly useful in identifying dementia in patients with cultural or language barriers and in differentiating between psychosis and dementia (Fink, Green, & Bender, 1952). The basis for the test is that people with organic disease tend to extinguish one or both of two sensations when touched simultaneously. In administering the test, the practitioner simultaneously touches the patient's cheek and palm over a period of 10 trials: 4 contra-lateral; 4 ipsi-lateral; and 2 symmetric stimuli interspersed. Prior to beginning the test, patients are told that they will be touched

**TABLE 11.4 The Mini-Mental State Examination**

| Maximum score | Orientation |
| --- | --- |
| 5 | What is the (year) (season) (date) (month)? |
| 5 | Where are we (state) (country) (hospital) (floor) (city)? |
| | Registration |
| 3 | Name three objects: One second to say each. Then ask the patient all three after you have said them. Give one point for each correct answer. Repeat them until he learns all three. Count trials and record number. |
| | ____Number of trials |
| | Attention and calculation |
| 5 | Begin with 100 and count backwards by 7 (stop after five answers). Alternatively, spell "world" backwards. |
| | Recall |
| 3 | Ask for the three objects repeated above. Give one point for each correct answer. |
| | Language |
| 2 | Show a pencil and a watch and ask subject to name them. |
| 1 | Repeat the following: "No ifs, ands, or buts." |
| 3 | A three-stage command, "Take a paper in your right hand; fold it in half, and put it on the floor." |
| 1 | Read and obey the following: (show subject the written item). |
| | CLOSE YOUR EYES |
| 1 | Write a sentence. |
| 1 | Copy a design (complex polygon as in Bender-Gestalt). |
| 30 | Total score possible |

*Note*. From "Mini-Mental State: A Practical Method for Grading the Cognitive State of Patients for the Clinician," by M.F. Folstein, S.E. Folstein, & P. McHugh, 1975, *Journal of Psychiatric Research*, *12*, pp. 189–198. Pergamon Press. Adapted by permission.

twice; the test can be conducted with the eyes open or closed. Only the last four of the ten paired tests, which follow the 2 symmetric stimuli, count toward the score. Dementia is suspected if patients score errors in the last 4 trials (Fink et al., 1952).

The increased fund of information and vocabulary that naturally occurs as one ages may cause tests solely based on verbal abilities to overestimate mental functioning. Early changes in mental and emotional functioning may be more clearly revealed by performance tests in

**TABLE 11.5 The Short Portable Mental Status Questionnaire (SPMSQ)**

1. What is the date today (month/day/year)? _/_/_
2. What day of the week is it? _____
3. What is the name of this place? _____
4. What is your telephone number? (If no telephone, what is your street address?) _____
5. How old are you? _____
6. When were you born (month/day/year)? _/_/_
7. Who is the current president of the United States? _____
8. Who was the president just before him? _____
9. What was your mother's maiden name? _____
10. Subtract 3 from 20 and keep subtracting each new number you get, all the way down.

0-2 errors  = intact
3-4 errors  = mild intellectual impairment
5-7 errors  = moderate intellectual impairment
8-10 errors = severe intellectual impairment

Allow one more error if subject had only grade school education.
Allow one fewer error if subject has had education beyond high school.
Allow one more error for blacks, regardless of education criteria.

*Note.* From "A Short Portable Mental Status Questionnaire for the Assessment of Organic Brain Deficit in Elderly Patients," by E. Pfeiffer, 1975, *Journal of the American Geriatrics Society, 23*, pp. 433–441. Reprinted with permission of the American Geriatrics Society.

which deficits tend to be more significant after age 65 (Weschler, 1955). Performance tests require hand-eye coordination, perceptual organization, and attention to detail and logical sequence. The MMS includes two performance items, writing one's name and copying a geometric form. Other types of performance tests that may be utilized include block design, object assembly, such as doing a simple jigsaw puzzle, and arranging pictures in sequence to tell a story (see Figure 11.1).

Instruments which measure cognition are not meant to be used in isolation but rather to round out a comprehensive picture of a person's mental health. These instruments are particularly useful in that they provide established "cut-off" scores that can trigger a suspicion of pathology, such as dementia, and lead to further, more specific testing. It is important to keep in mind, however, that low or abnormal scores on mental status tests do not differentiate among specific diagnoses. The full history and physical examination, along with laboratory tests, are needed to determine a specific diagnosis, for example, to differentiate between delirium or dementia.

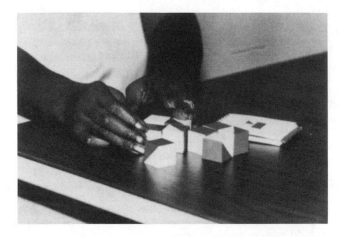

**FIGURE 11.1. Performance test using block designs to determine abstract intellectual function.**

## Affective Disorders: Depression

Only about 5% of community-residing elderly evidence symptomatic depression which meets the Diagnostic and Statistical Manual of Mental Disorders, Third Edition, Revised, (DSM III-R) criteria for clinical depression. But close to 20% of older people report depressive symptoms (Blazer, 1989). Such symptoms may be mild and frequently occur as a reactive depression secondary to grief and bereavement, loss of social contacts and social isolation, or physical illness. People with chronic obstructive pulmonary disease, for example, are thought to be particularly vulnerable to depression.

The DSM III-R criteria for clinical depression are shown in Table 11.6. Unfortunately, these criteria fail to adequately address some of the physical, functional, and social losses which so frequently contribute to or compound the reactive depression of old age. While manifestations of depression are the same as in any age group, nearly 20% of elderly people with depression present with somatic complaints of physical illness such as weight loss, low energy level, poor appetite, and sleep disturbances (Gottleib, 1989). Psychomotor retardation, extreme lethargy, and ruminations focused on negative thoughts and death are common. When severe, symptoms may mimic dementia, a condition known as pseudodementia. An agitated depression, on the other hand, is characterized by symptoms such as pacing, vocalizations, and hand wringing.

## TABLE 11.6 The DSM-III-R Criteria for Clinical Depression

1. Depressed mood most of the time, as indicated by looking and feeling sad, hopeless, and/or discouraged.
2. Markedly diminished interest or pleasure in all or most activities—apathy, withdrawal, not caring.
3. Significant weight loss or weight gain.
4. Insomnia or hypersomnia—difficulty sleeping or sleeping too much.
5. Fatigue or loss of energy.
6. Feelings of worthlessness, low self-esteem, or inappropriate guilt.
7. Diminished ability to think or to concentrate, or difficulty making decisions.
8. Psychomotor agitation or retardation—excessive activity, usually nonpro-ductive and repetitious, or slowing of physical reactions, movements, and speech.
9. Recurrent thoughts of death, thoughts of suicide, or suicide attempt.

*Note.* From the American Psychiatric Association, *Diagnostic and Statistical Manual of Mental Disorders, Third Edition, Revised,* Washington, DC: American Psychiatric Association, 1987. Reprinted with permission.

It is important to ascertain if the client's despondent outlook and behavior are recent changes or represent a lifelong pattern of behavior. Since mortality in the year following death of a spouse increases sevenfold, the practitioner should ascertain from clients whether exacerbation of symptoms, for example, increase of vague somatic complaints or avoidance of friends and customary social events, coincides with the death or the anniversary of the death of a loved one, referred to as the "anniversary phenomenon."

Of added concern with depression in older people is the high suicide risk in the elderly. Although the aged comprise only 12% of the total population, 25% of successful suicides occur in people 65 and over. The suicide rate in white males over 65 is four times the national average, and in white females over 65 it is two times the national average (U.S. National Center for Health Statistics, 1986).

Several objective scales specifically assess depression. Among the most frequently used is The Yesavage Geriatric Depression Scale (Table 11.7). This scale contains 30 clinically derived items to which clients can answer "yes" or "no" directly or by having the items read to them (Yesavage et al., 1983). The items, 20 of which are positive and 10 of which are negative, yield a score of 0 (no depression) to 30 (very depressed). A score of greater than 10 indicates possible depression. The Yesavage Scale is easy to administer and has been used extensively with community-residing elderly (Yesavage et al., 1983).

**TABLE 11.7 The Yesavage Geriatric Depression Scale**

Choose the best answer for how you felt over the past week.

| | |
|---|---|
| 1. Are you basically satisfied with your life? | yes/no |
| 2. Have you dropped many of your activities and interests? | yes/no |
| 3. Do you feel that your life is empty? | yes/no |
| 4. Do you often get bored? | yes/no |
| 5. Are you hopeful about the future? | yes/no |
| 6. Are you bothered by thoughts that you can't get out of your head? | yes/no |
| 7. Are you in good spirits most of the time? | yes/no |
| 8. Are you afraid that something bad is going to happen to you? | yes/no |
| 9. Do you feel happy most of the time? | yes/no |
| 10. Do you often feel helpless? | yes/no |
| 11. Do you often get restless and fidgety? | yes/no |
| 12. Do you prefer to stay at home, rather than going out doing new things? | yes/no |
| 13. Do you frequently worry about the future? | yes/no |
| 14. Do you feel you have more problems with your memory than most? | yes/no |
| 15. Do you think it is wonderful to be alive now? | yes/no |
| 16. Do you often feel downhearted and blue? | yes/no |
| 17. Do you feel pretty worthless the way you are now? | yes/no |
| 18. Do you worry a lot about the past? | yes/no |
| 19. Do you find life very exciting? | yes/no |
| 20. Is it hard for you to get started on new projects? | yes/no |
| 21. Do you feel full of energy? | yes/no |
| 22. Do you feel that your situation is hopeless? | yes/no |
| 23. Do you think that most people are better off than you are? | yes/no |
| 24. Do you frequently get upset over little things? | yes/no |
| 25. Do you frequently feel like crying? | yes/no |
| 26. Do you have trouble concentrating? | yes/no |
| 27. Do you enjoy getting up in the morning? | yes/no |
| 28. Do you prefer to avoid social gatherings? | yes/no |
| 29. Is it easy for you to make decisions? | yes/no |
| 30. Is your mind as clear as it used to be? | yes/no |

Note. From "Development and Validation of a Geriatric Depression Screening Scale: A Preliminary Report", by J. Yesavage et al., 1983, *Journal of Psychiatric Research, 17*, pp. 37–49. @ 1983, Pergamon Press. Reprinted with permission.

## Dementia Assessment

Approximately 10% of people 65 and over residing in the community, as many as 45% of community-residing elderly age 85 and over, and 60% of people in long-term care facilities are thought to have dementia (Gottleib, 1989). Alzheimer's disease (AD), the most common form of dementia, remains a clinical diagnosis. There is no single sign or unique pattern of impairment, and no laboratory test or imaging technique which can conclusively detect AD. The diagnosis is made following a careful history and physical examination by ruling out other possible causes of symptoms, and by following people over time.

Criteria for a presumptive diagnosis of AD are shown in Table 11.8. To make a probable diagnosis of AD, the patient must be between the ages of 40 and 90 (most often 65 or older) and exhibit an abnormal score on a mental status instrument, two or more areas of cognitive deficits, and progressive worsening of memory, first recent memory and subsequently remote memory, as well as other cognitive functions (American Geriatrics Society, 1985). Memory for "landmark" events may be less subject to forgetting than memory for transient events (Fromholt & Larsen, 1991).

**TABLE 11.8 Criteria for Clinical Diagnosis of Alzheimer's Disease**

---

I. The criteria for the clinical diagnosis of PROBABLE Alzheimer's disease include:

dementia established by clinical examination and documented by the Mini-Mental Test, Blessed Dementia Scale, or some similar examination, and confirmed by neuropsychological tests;

deficits in two or more areas of cognition;

progressive worsening of memory and other cognitive functions;

no disturbance of consciousness;

onset between ages 40 and 90, most often after age 65; and

absence of systemic disorders or other brain diseases that in and of themselves could account for the progressive deficits in memory and cognition.

II. The diagnosis of PROBABLE Alzheimer's disease is supported by:

progressive deterioration of specific cognitive functions such as language (aphasia), motor skills (apraxia), and perception (agnosia);

impaired activities of daily living and altered patterns of behavior;

family history of similar disorders, particularly if confirmed neuropathologically; and

laboratory results of:

normal lumbar puncture as evaluated by standard techniques,

normal pattern or nonspecific changes in EEG, such as increased slow-wave activity, and

evidence of cerebral atrophy on CT with progression documented by serial observation.

III. Other clinical features consistent with the diagnosis of PROBABLE Alzheimer's disease, after exclusion of causes of dementia other than Alzheimer's disease, include:

plateaus in the course of progression of the illness;

associated symptoms of depression, insomnia, incontinence, delusions, illusions, hallucinations, catastrophic verbal, emotional, or physical out-bursts, sexual disorders, and weight loss;

*(continued)*

other neurologic abnormalities in some patients, especially with more
advanced disease and including motor signs such as increased muscle
tone, myoclonus, or gait disorder;
seizures in advanced disease; and
CT normal for age.

IV. Features that make the diagnosis of PROBABLE Alzheimer's disease uncertain or unlikely include:
sudden, apoplectic onset;
focal neurologic findings such as hemiparesis, sensory loss, visual field
deficits, and incoordination early in the course of the illness; and
seizures or gait disturbances at the onset or very early in the course of
the illness.

V. Clinical diagnosis of POSSIBLE Alzheimer's disease:
may be made on the basis of the dementia syndrome, in the absence of
other neurologic, psychiatric, or systemic disorders sufficient to cause
dementia, and in the presence of variations in the onset, in the
presentation, or in the clinical course;
may be made in the presence of a second systemic or brain disorder
sufficient to produce dementia, which is not considered to be the cause
of the dementia; and
should be used in research studies when a single, gradually progressive
severe cognitive deficit is identified in the absence of other identifiable
cause.

VI. Criteria for diagnosis of DEFINITE Alzheimer's disease are:
the clinical criteria for probable Alzheimer's disease and
histopathologic evidence obtained from a biopsy or autopsy.

VII. Classification of Alzheimer's disease for research purposes should specify
features that may differentiate subtypes of the disorder, such as:
familial occurrence;
onset before age 65;
presence of trisomy-21; and
coexistence of other relevant conditions such as Parkinson's disease.

---

*Note.* From "Criteria for the Clinical Diagnosis of Alzheimer's Disease: Excerpts from the
NINCDS-ADRDA Work Group Report." *Journal of the American Geriatrics Society, 33,* 244–
250. Reprinted with permission of the American Geriatrics Society.

A presumptive diagnosis of AD requires that there be no disturbance
of consciousness, no systemic disorders, and no other brain diseases.
A diagnosis of AD cannot be made when consciousness is impaired or
when other clinical abnormalities prevent adequate evaluation of mental
status (American Geriatrics Society, 1985). The predominant early signs
and symptoms of dementia, which the practitioner will observe during the assessment, include decrease in recent memory, decreased
ability to comprehend directions, and diminished ability for abstract
reasoning and computation. Later symptoms include disorientation to
time and place, inappropriate affect, and loss of judgment shown by

inappropriate dress and social behavior (American Geriatrics Society, 1985; Reisberg, Ferris, & Franssen, 1985).

As many as 16% of dementias are potentially reversible. When dementia is first suspected, a systematic workup should be undertaken to rule out reversible causes. Referral to a specialized dementia center may be warranted. The Dementia Acronym (Table 11.9), developed by Dietrich, includes the parameters of such an assessment (Deitrich, 1989). Drug toxicity, the most common primary cause of reversible dementia, accounts for approximately 2.7% of all cases of dementia and often compounds the symptoms of an underlying dementia (Morrison

**TABLE 11.9 Dementia Acronym**

D  Drugs
    Psychotropics
    Polypharmacy
E  Emotional distress
    Depression
    Stress
    Bereavement
M  Metabolic/endocrine disorders
    Diabetes
    Hypothyroidism
    Dehydration
E  Environment/eyes/ears
    Changes in living situation
    Sensory losses
N  Nutritional
    Anemia, B12, Folic acid
    Alcoholism
    Constipation
    Anorexia
    Poor dentition
    Self-starvation
    Inability to purchase food
    Depression
T  Tumors
    Trauma
I  Infections
    Pneumonia
    Urinary tract
A  Acute illness
    Congestive Heart Failure
    Myocardial infarction
    Pulmonary Emboli

*Note.* From *Caring for the Psychogeriatric Client* (p. 111) by C. Deitrich in P. Ebersole, 1989. New York: Springer Publishing Company, Inc. Used by permission.

& Katz, 1989). Drugs most frequently implicated are those with anti-cholinergic properties, sedative hypnotics, analgesics, antihypertensives, and H-2 receptor antagonists, particularly cimetadine. These medications cause both overt and subclinical symptoms, which may only be detected using standardized assessment measures. Taking four or more prescription medications markedly increases the risk for drug-related impairment.

Progression and worsening of symptoms is critical to the diagnosis of AD. Reisberg and associates (1985) have identified seven distinguishable stages of AD:

1) no cognitive decline
2) very mild cognitive decline (forgetfulness phase)
3) mild cognitive decline (early confusional phase)
4) moderate cognitive decline (late confusional phase)
5) moderately severe cognitive decline (early dementia phase)
6) severe cognitive decline (mid-dementia phase)
7) very severe cognitive decline (late dementia phase)

AD can only be diagnosed with relative certainty during the fourth stage (Reisberg et al., 1985).

Multi-infarct Dementia (MID) is differentiated from AD primarily by history and laboratory confirmation of vascular disease such as hypertension and cerebral vascular accidents. There is often a more abrupt onset and stepwise progression, and presence of focal neurological findings such as spasticity and superbulbar palsy. A careful history is especially helpful in differentiating between AD and MID.

## Delirium Assessment

Delirium is an organic brain syndrome characterized by global cognitive impairment of abrupt onset and relatively brief duration (usually less than a month) associated with disturbances of attention, sleep-wake cycle, and psychomotor behavior (Lipowski, 1989). In contrast to dementia, delirium has a rapid onset, a fluctuating course, and is of brief duration, lasting no more than 2 or 3 weeks. The term delirium is often used synonymously with confusion, disorientation, or acute confusional state. Because it is more clearly and precisely defined, delirium is accepted as the more accurate of these terms. The incidence of delirium in hospitalized elderly is thought to be between 20% and 30% (Lipowski, 1989; Johnson, Gottleib, Sullivan et al., 1990; Sullivan, Wanich, & Kurlowicz, 1991).

While no instruments specifically screen for delirium, the DSM III-R lists specific criteria which must be present for a presumptive diagnosis of delirium (Table 11.10). Disorientation and memory impairment are only two of many presenting symptoms, although delirious patients are rarely disoriented as to person. The most common additional presenting features are:

1) attention disorders demonstrated by altered alertness, distractibility and inability to concentrate
2) disorganized thought as evidenced by rambling, irrelevant, or incoherent speech
3) behavioral manifestations including disturbance of sleep-wake cycle, daytime drowsiness, insomnia, disturbing dreams, nightmares or hallucinations, and reduced or heightened psychomotor activity and responsiveness, such as anxiety and restlessness (Lipowski, 1989; Johnson et al., 1990).

Symptoms often fluctuate between periods of disturbed responses and more lucid periods.

As in dementia, drug toxicity is the most common cause of delirium. The drugs mentioned previously as the primary or secondary cause of dementia are also those implicated as causative agents of delirium (Deitrich, 1989). Delirium may also herald the onset of an organic illness, such as infection.

## Differentiation Between Pseudodementia, Dementia, Delirium, and Depression

Symptoms which older people construe to be evidence of dementia may, in fact, reflect commonly occurring and benign manifestations of

---

**TABLE 11.10 Criteria for Presumptive Diagnosis of Delirium**

1. Reduced ability to maintain attention to external stimuli; distractibility, with the need to have questions repeated.
2. Disorganized thinking, as indicated by rambling, irrelevant, or incoherent speech.
3. Reduced level of consciousness, with difficulty of arousal or staying awake.
4. Illusions, hallucinations, or other perceptual disturbance.
5. Disorientation to person, place, or time.
6. Memory impairment.
7. Disturbance of the sleep-wake cycle, with insomnia at night or daytime sleepiness.
8. Increased or decreased psychomotor activity, with either agitation and restlessness or generalized slowing of movement and speech.

*Note.* From *Diagnostic and Statistical Manual of Mental Disorders, Third Edition, Revised.* 1987. Washington, DC: American Psychiatric Association. Reprinted with permission.

aging, or may be caused by conditions other than dementia. Delayed or impaired recall of recent events, sometimes called benign senile forgetfulness, is very common in the elderly and does not constitute dementia.

The major differentiating factors between dementia, depression (pseudodementia), and delirium are shown in Table 11.11. Pseudodementia refers to a cluster of symptoms which mimic dementia but which, on careful exploration, have an identifiable cause. The most common cause is depression in the absence of, or in conjunction with, a true dementia. Diagnosis of depression as the cause of a pseudodementia must often await the patient's response to antidepressant medications. Drug toxicity and chronic illnesses, such as hypothyroidism, can also cause symptoms of a pseudodementia.

In contrast to dementia and depression, the onset of symptoms of delirium is acute and characterized by anxiety, restlessness, and alterations in level of consciousness, such as drowsiness. Cognitive functioning is impaired but symptoms wax and wane, with episodes of lucidity interspersed with loss of contact with reality and/or psychotic behavior such as hallucinations (Francis, Martin, & Kapoor, 1990). Psychomotor behavior can fluctuate unpredictably between hypoactivity and hyperactivity (Lipowski, 1989).

In evaluating confused, disoriented, or demented elderly clients, it is important to verify their response patterns and specific answers to questions with people who know them well, such as family, friends, or companions. Severity of mental impairment has also been shown to correlate with deficits in functional ability (Goldfarb, 1974).

The practitioner should keep in mind that apathy of response may represent depression or withdrawal from an oppressive situation rather than a deterioration of mental functioning. The apparent indifference may also be used as a cover-up as in the case when the client is aware of failing mental capacities and thus tries to conceal the fact that he or she is unable to respond correctly.

## IMPLICATIONS FOR PRACTICE

There is a significant primary prevention role with regard to the mental/emotional status of the older client. Practitioners should support a positive self-image and encourage older people to pursue a variety of interests and involvement in social activities. Encouraging older people to establish close relationships can help create linkages with people and services which are potential sources for social support. Helping clients to modify risk factors such as stress, social isola-

**TABLE 11.11 Differentiation Between Dementia, Depression (Pseudodementia), and Delirium**

| Parameter | Dementia | Depression | Delirium |
|---|---|---|---|
| Onset | Months to years | Weeks | Short/rapid Abrupt Hours/days |
| Duration | 5 to 15 years | 3 to 6 months May be chronic | Days to 3 weeks |
| Initial presentation | Vague symptoms Loss of intellect Denies/conceals symptoms Easily distracted Great effort to perform tasks | Flat affect Hypochondriasis Focuses on symptoms Apathy Little effort to perform tasks | Disorientation Clouded consciousness Fluctuated Moods Disordered thoughts Fails to understand tasks |
| Recent memory | Impaired; Perseveration Confabulation | Normal or recent/past both altered | Patchy Remote intact |
| Intellect | Impaired Concrete thinking | Slowed; may be unwilling to respond | Impaired |
| Judgment | Impaired; Bad/ inappropriate decisions Denies problem | Poor judgment Many "don't know" answers | Impaired Difficulty separating facts & hallucinations |
| Diurnal Pattern | Worse in evening "Sundowning" Reversed sleep | Worse in morning; Sleep impaired | Day drowsiness Nighttime hallucinations; Insomnia; Nightmares |
| Attention | Easily distracted | Withdrawn | Labile |
| Affect | Shallow; Labile; Inappropriate anxiety; Depression Suspicious | Constricted Apathy Hopeless Distressed | Variable Fear/panic Euphoria Disturbed |
| Orientation | Disoriented | Intact | Disoriented, but usually not to person Periods of lucidity |
| Level of consciousness | Intact | Intact | Disturbed |
| Psychotic symptoms | Late Delusions Hallucinations | Delusions | Delusions |

*Note.* From *Clinical Internal Medicine in the Aged*, by R. Schrier, 1982, Philadelphia: W.B. Saunders Co. *Caring for the Psychogeriatric Client*, by P. Ebersole, 1989. New York: Springer Publishing Co. "A comprehensive view of delirium in the elderly," by Z.J. Lipowski, 1986, *Geriatric Consultant* March/April. "Optimizing Mental Function of the Elderly," by G. Gottleib In *Practicing Prevention for the Elderly* (pp. 153–166) by R. Lavizzo-Mourey, S. Day, D. Diserens and J.A. Grisso (Eds.), 1989, Philadelphia: Hanley & Belfus, Inc.

tion, and substance abuse is an important primary prevention strategy. Nurses can help older clients appreciate the extent to which their emotional status affects their ability to adapt to changes in health and to life crises common to aging. Older people should be encouraged to use previous patterns of appropriate adaptive behavior to meet current life crises.

Secondary prevention focuses on encouraging older people to seek health screening for early signs and symptoms of mental health changes, and on case finding. Providers need to take a positive approach to the mental health needs of the elderly. Of great importance is assuring a correct diagnosis, which often includes differentiating between depression, delirium and dementia, including identifying potentially reversible causes of dementia. It is important to keep in mind that mental deterioration is often the first sign of an organic physical illness. For example, sudden confusion or apathy in an older person may be the first observable sign of an acute infectious process such as pneumonia.

Tertiary prevention offers opportunities to provide ongoing support and management for mental health problems. Management of depression in older clients is an important area for intervention, especially given its severity and the high risk for suicide among the depressed elderly. Referral for psychiatric evaluation, development of support groups, individual counseling, and the recognition of the need for special attention at the time of anniversaries of painful losses may be helpful interventions.

If dementia is suspected, a complete history and mental/emotional status examination are essential in assessing the cause and severity of the impairment. It is important to differentiate between mental status changes that are manifestations of a reversible toxic or metabolic psychosis and those which result from a degenerative process in the central nervous system. Such an assessment often requires referral to a center specifically organized to perform comprehensive, interdisciplinary evaluations for dementia. When a diagnosis of a true dementia, such as Alzheimer's disease, is confirmed, the comprehensive assessment provides the basis for therapeutic plans which focus on preserving the older client's functional capabilities at an optimum level and in assisting patients and families to anticipate, cope with, and plan for the evolving behavioral changes.

## REFERENCES

American Geriatrics Society. (1985). Criteria for the clinical diagnosis of Alzheimer's disease: Excerpts from the NINCDS-ADRDA Work Group Report. *Journal of the American Geriatrics Society, 33*, 244–250.

Blazer, D. (1989). Depression in late life: An update. In Lawton, P. (Ed.), *Annual review of geriatrics and gerontology* (pp. 197–214). New York: Springer Publishing Co.

Deitrich, C. (1989). In Ebersole, P. *Caring for the psychogeriatric client* (p. 111). New York: Springer Publishing Co.

Fink, M., Green, M., & Bender, M. B. (1952). The face-hand test as a diagnostic sign of organic mental syndrome. *Neurology, 2,* 46–59.

Folstein, M. F., Folstein, S. E., & McHugh, P. (1975). Mini-mental state: A practical method for grading the cognitive state of patients for the clinician. *Journal of Psychiatric Research, 12,* 189–98.

Francis, J., Martin, D., & Kapoor, W. (1990). A prospective study of delirium in hospitalized elderly. *Journal of the American Medical Association, 263,* 1097–1101.

Fromholt, P., & Larsen, S. (1991). Autobiographical memory in normal aging and primary degenerative dementia (dementia of Alzheimer's type). *Journal of Gerontology, 46,* 85–91.

Goldfarb, A. I. (1974). *Aging and the organic brain syndrome* (pp. 11–13). Washington, PA: McNeil Laboratories.

Gordon, S., & Stokes, S. (1988). Development of an instrument to measure stress in the older adult. *Nursing Research, 37,* 34–8.

Gottlieb, G. (1989). Optimizing mental function of the elderly. In Lavizzo-Mourey, R., Day, S., Diserens, D., & Grisso, J. A. (Eds.), *Practicing prevention for the elderly* (pp. 153–166). Philadelphia: Hanley & Belfus, Inc.

Johnson, J., Gottlieb, G., Sullivan, E., et al. (1990). Using DSM III criteria to diagnose delirium in elderly general medical patients. *Journals of Gerontology, 45,* M113–19.

Kane, R. A., & Kane, R. L. (1988). *Assessing the elderly: A practical guide to measurement.* Lexington, MA: Lexington Books.

Lipowski, Z. J. (1989). Delirium in the elderly patients. *New England Journal of Medicine, 320,* 578–582.

Morrison, R., & Katz, I. (1989). Drug-related cognitive impairment: Current progress and recurrent problems. In Lawton, P. (Ed.), *Annual review of gerontology and geriatrics* (pp. 232–279). New York: Springer Publishing Co.

Newman, S., Struyk, R., Wright, P., & Rice, M. (1990). Overwhelming odds: Caregiving and the risk of institutionalization. *Journals of Gerontology, 45,* S173–183.

Pfeiffer, E. (1975). A short portable mental status questionnaire for the assessment of organic brain deficit in elderly patients. *Journal of the American Geriatrics Society, 23,* 433–441.

Reisberg, B., Ferris, S., & Franssen, E. (1985). An ordinal functional assessment tool for Alzheimer's type dementia. *Hospital and Community Psychiatry, 36,* 593–595.

Sullivan, E., Wanich, C., & Kurlowicz, L. (1991). Nursing assessment and management of delirium in the elderly. *American Operating Room Nurses (AORN) Journal, 53,* 820–828.

U.S. National Center for Health Statistics. (1986). *Vital statistics of the United States, annual.* Washington, DC: U.S. Government Printing Office.

Weschler, D. (1955). *Manual for the Weschler Adult Intelligence Scale* (pp. 82, 92, 103, 108, 110). New York: Psychological Corporation.

Yesavage, J. et al. (1983). Development and validation of a geriatric depression screening scale: A preliminary report. *Journal of Psychiatric Research, 17,* 37–49.

## SUGGESTED READINGS

Abraham, I., & Neundorfer, M. (1990). Alzheimer's: A decade of progress, a future of nursing challenges. *Geriatric Nursing, 11,* 116–19.

American Psychiatric Association. (1986). Diagnostic and Statistical Manual DSM III-R. Washington, DC: Author.

Chenitz, C., Stone, J., & Salisbury, S. (1991). *Clinical gerontological nursing: A guide to advanced practice.* Philadelphia: W.B. Saunders Co.

Ebersole, P. (1989). *Caring for the psychogeriatric client.* New York: Springer Publishing Co.

Eliopolous, C. (1990). *Health assessment of the older adult,* (Second Edition). Redwood City, CA: Addison-Wesley Nursing; A Division of The Benjamin/ Cummings Publishing Company Inc.

Evans, D., Funkenstein, H., Albert, M., Scherr, P., Cook, N., Chown, M., Hebert, L., Hennekens, C., & Taylor, J. (1989). Prevalence of Alzheimer's disease in a community population of older persons. *Journal of the American Medical Association, 262,* 2551–2556.

Fulmer, T., & Walker, M. (1991). *Critical care nursing of the elderly.* Springer Services on Geriatric Nursing. New York: Springer Publishing Co.

Kane, R. A., & Kane, R. L. (1988). *Assessing the elderly: A practical guide to measurement.* Lexington, MA: Lexington Books.

Lavizzo-Mourey, R., Day, S., Diserens, D., & Grisso, J. A. (1989). *Practicing Prevention for the Elderly* (pp. 153–166). Philadelphia: Hanley & Belfus, Inc.

Lipowski, Z. J. (1987). Delirium (acute confusional states). *Journal of the American Medical Association, 258,* 1789–1792.

# 12

# Assessment of Neurological Functioning

Despite numerous age-related changes in the nervous system (for example, loss of neurons and brain mass, decreased nerve condition velocity, and increased reflex response times), most older people do not manifest significant or observable changes in cognition, motor coordination, or behavior unless a neurological disease is present. Healthy older persons, however, are more susceptible to transitory central nervous system-related drug side effects and are more likely to have signs and symptoms of brain hypoxia with medical illnesses such as anemia, heart failure, or pneumonia (Joynt, 1990).

Careful neurological assessment is crucial given the frequent occurrence of primary neurologic diseases in older persons, as well as the common expression of other illnesses through secondary dysfunction in the nervous system (Besdine, 1990). Neurological disorders remain a leading cause of institutionalization and altered lifestyle in this age group (Gambert, 1987, p. 323). The neurological diseases that occur most commonly in this age group are the degenerative and cerebrovascular disorders. Epilepsy, muscular dystrophies, and demyelinating disorders are not characteristic. The elderly may develop other neurological disorders that occur at any age (such as brain tumors and central nervous system infections), but they tend to have different manifestations, treatment, and prognosis in the elderly; for example, seizures in the elderly are more likely to be the result of a structural abnormality, such as a brain tumor (Joynt, 1990, p. 926). The neurological history of older persons

159

focuses on exploring presented symptoms and seeking information related to the neurological disorders for which they are particularly at risk.

# HISTORY

## Client Profile

In the client profile section of the health history, the practitioner elicits data descriptive of habits that increase the risk of strokes (such as overeating, high sodium and/or cholesterol diet, smoking, or ineffective stress management) as well as the use of substances (alcohol or other drugs) that alter central nervous system functioning. In addition, chronic nutritional inadequacies that can impair neurological functioning may be revealed.

## Past Health History

Neurological assessment of the older client begins with exploration of any past neurological diseases, injuries, or symptoms, as well as evidence of current symptomatology related to the most prevalent neurological disorders in the older population: transient ischemic attacks (TIAs), stroke, Parkinson's disease, intracranial tumors, and peripheral neuropathies (which may be caused by herpes zoster, diabetes, nutritional disorders, and/or alcoholism). Infectious diseases of the central nervous system are of particular concern because of their high rates of morbidity and mortality in the elderly. In addition, if there is evidence of increased mental confusion and/or decreased mental awareness, reversible causes of delirium (for example, acute illness, medication use, and/or sensory deficits) need to be distinguished from irreversible dementia (Burrage, 1991, pp. 82–83). (For a more complete discussion, see Chapter 11, Assessment of Mental/Emotional Status.)

Significant data indicating a higher level of risk for stroke would include a history of:

1. hypertension, especially if severe and poorly controlled
2. cardiac arrhythmias
3. transient ischemic attacks
4. arteriosclerotic disease (cardiac or peripheral)
5. diabetes mellitus
6. valvular heart disease
7. surgical implantation of a prosthetic heart valve
8. polycythemia

Central nervous system pathology and functional changes in the older client may also result from a history of chronic alcoholism, malnutrition, or untreated syphilis that progresses to the tertiary stage. History of infectious diseases that sometimes have neurological sequelae (such as influenza or encephalitis) may be significant.

Questions should also be asked about cardiac or respiratory conditions that may decrease cerebral oxygenation and, thus, cause syncope, confusion, or other mental status changes in the older person. These conditions include congestive heart failure, bradycardia, heart block (Stokes-Adams Syndrome), and pulmonary emphysema. As at any age, a past history of central nervous system trauma or surgery is relevant.

The history includes data concerning drugs that the client has taken in the past or is presently taking. Examples of medications that would be considered especially pertinent to this area of assessment include:

1. drugs that may cause signs and symptoms of Parkinsonism, such as the phenothiazines
2. central nervous system stimulants or depressants
3. tranquilizers, mood elevators, and other drugs that may alter mood and affect (for example, corticosteroids)
4. anticoagulants, which may predispose to cerebral hemorrhage
5. antihypertensives or drugs that slow the heart rate (for example, digitalis preparations) and may decrease cerebral perfusion.

## Review of Systems

Sections of the review of systems relevant to assessment of this area of functioning include not only the neurologic segment but also many symptoms usually classified under other systems—for example, changes in vision, hearing, equilibrium, speech, and bowel and bladder control.

Because the elderly may experience transient fluctuations in alertness or amnesic episodes in relation to transient ischemic attacks (TIAs) or small vessel strokes, it is important to carefully question older clients about any periods of decreased alertness, lethargy, somnolence, disorientation, or amnesia.

If the older client complains of headache, it is important to obtain a detailed description of the onset, quality, severity, location, temporal characteristics, and precipitating and aggravating/relieving factors. Tension headaches are common, but arthritis of the cervical spine, cerebrovascular disease, uncontrolled hypertension (>180/110 mmHg), brain tumors, subdural hematoma (subsequent to falls), trigeminal neuralgia, temporomandibular joint (TMJ) syndrome, and temporal arteritis are more serious causes of head pain in older adults. Although migraine headaches are rare in elderly individuals, cluster headaches may occur in the 7th decade (Burrage, 1991, pp. 83–84).

Specific review of neurologic symptoms will also include eliciting any changes in motor strength or coordination of the upper or lower extremities and their effect on the client's gait or ability to engage in activities of daily living. If the older client complains of unsteadiness, clumsiness or dizziness, a history of previous head injury, episodic vertigo, and cranial nerve symptoms may indicate a neurological problem rather than inner ear disease (Bonikowski, 1983). A number of neurologic conditions are commonly associated with falls in the elderly, including Parkinson's disease, normal-pressure hydrocephalus, seizure disorders, cerebellar lesions and drop attacks (Stone & Chenitz, 1991). "Drop attacks" are characterized by a sudden buckling of the legs, without loss of consciousness, due to a transitory loss of muscle tone and strength in the lower extremities. If reported, the practitioner should determine if the client is aware of the impending fall and has sufficient time to initiate safety precautions. Syncopal attacks, on the other hand, are always accompanied by loss of consciousness and can occur in the elderly following hot baths or initiation of the Valsalva maneuver.

An older client's report of motor weakness may be due to movement disorders resulting from disease of the cerebral cortex, cerebellum, or basal ganglia, primary motor neuron disease, or peripheral neuropathy. However, other medical conditions such as diminished cardiac reserve, inflammatory arthritis, or primary muscle disease may also cause weakness. It is important to ascertain the specific location and extent of the weakness, as well as specific activities that have alerted the older client to this symptom (for example, lifting, rising from chair or bed, or stair climbing).

Any changes in sensation noted by the client may be evidence of underlying disease. Therefore, they should also be carefully elicited and described.

## PHYSICAL EXAMINATION

### Overview

The neurologic examination is more difficult to accomplish with the older person because many clients have more difficulty in cooperating with the various components of the complete neurologic exam, particularly the sensory exam. The client is asked to follow many commands and tends to tire more easily than a younger client. Demonstration by the examiner of the performance task being tested may be helpful. It is also helpful to spend time reassuring the older client and gaining his or her confidence.

It may be necessary to do the total neurologic examination at a separate time from the rest of the physical examination, so that the client is not overfatigued. Or it may be preferable to do selected aspects of the examination over several sessions. Retesting may be necessary to validate results. In each part of the examination, the practitioner should allow for a longer reaction time after presenting each stimulus than would be the case with a younger adult.

The major changes in the nervous system associated with the aging process are: a progressive decrease in the number of functioning neurons in the central nervous system and sense organs; and a slowing of the speed of impulse transmission and reaction to stimuli. Because of the tremendous reserves in the number and capacity of the brain cells, the older person usually functions well despite the progressive loss of neurons. Those in the upper 5% of mental ability often show very little change with advancing age. However, older persons generally show some degree of impairment of hearing, vision, smell, temperature and pain sensation, memory, and mental endurance, as well as a lengthening of their reaction time. Although, in the absence of disease, healthy older adults demonstrate little change in the function of information storage, they do experience a loss of speed in learning and processing new information and in reacting to simple or complex stimuli (Katzman & Terry, 1983).

## Cranial Nerves

Testing for cranial nerve function and the changes common in the elderly have been discussed in Chapter 6. Table 12.1 summarizes adaptations in examination techniques and common changes in cranial nerve function that are relevant to assessment of the older client. In general, the practitioner should allow a longer time for response when eliciting cranial nerve function than would be required for a younger adult.

## Motor Function

Examination of motor function includes inspection of muscle bulk, palpation of muscle tone, and testing of muscle strength against resistance. Even in the active older client there is usually a symmetrical decrease in muscle bulk, particularly in the dorsal interosseous muscle between the thumb and hand (Locke & Galabarda, 1978) and in the thigh and calf muscles (Shaumberg, Spencer, & Ochoa, 1983). When relaxed muscles are palpated, most older people show some decrease in muscle tone; however, there is often increased tone on passive

**TABLE 12.1 Differences in Cranial Nerve Assessment Techniques and Findings in the Older Client**

| Cranial nerve | Common changes in the elderly | Adaptations in test techniques |
|---|---|---|
| 1. Olfactory | Progressive loss of smell | None |
| 2. Optic | Decreased visual acuity | Use brighter light and place light source behind client |
| | Presbyopia | Diminished peripheral vision when testing for visual acuity. |
| | Fundoscopic changes: arteriolar narrowing of vessels | |
| | Increased tortuosity and silver-wire appearance of arterioles | |
| | Retinal pallor | |
| | Pupils smaller, with less brisk reaction to light and accommodation; may be unequal in size or irregular in shape | |
| 3. Oculomotor | No expected changes in extraocular eye movements | None |
| 4. Trochlear | | |
| 5. Abducens | | |
| 6. Trigeminal | None | None |
| 7. Facial | | |
|    Sensory: | Decreased perception of all taste modalities, especially sweet and salt | Need to use concentrated solution since threshold is raised. |
|    Motor: | May be facial asymmetry in edentulous client unrelated to facial nerve function. | Test with dentures in place. |
| 8. Auditory | | |
|    Presbycusis | Initially increase in loss of high tones. | Test in a very quiet environment. |
| | Later, loss generalized to all frequencies. | |
| 9. Glossopharyngeal | Gag reflex should be present; may be sluggish | |
| 10. Vagus | None | None |
| 11. Spinal accessory | None | None |
| 12. Hypoglossal | None | None |

movement. This involuntary rigidity should not be mistaken for lack of cooperation (Gallo, Reichel, & Andersen, 1988). Muscle tone of elderly individuals is also often difficult to assess because rigidity may be caused by joint disorders as well as neuromuscular disease. If muscle tone seems increased, the examiner should put the limb passively through its entire range of motion while palpating the muscle. This will help to differentiate spasticity or hypertonia, in which resistance is maximal on initial movement, from joint stiffness or Parkinson's syndrome, with "lead-pipe" rigidity throughout the range of motion or cogwheel rigidity in which the tremor periodically releases the muscle tension and creates a rhythmic, rachet-like resistance. Gegenhalten (continued fluctuation of resistance in a muscle during passive range of motion, despite efforts to gain the client's cooperation and relaxation) is seen in degenerative central nervous system disorders such as Alzheimer's disease (Adams & Victor, 1989).

The older person usually has some decrease in muscle strength that should correlate with the degree of decrease in muscle bulk. The strength of hand grips should be reasonably well-preserved, despite wasting of the fine muscles of the hands. After age 70 there is less difference in strength between the dominant and non-dominant hand than in the younger person. Rapid decrease in strength, or significant differences in symmetry of muscle strength, are abnormal and should be referred.

Evaluation of the older client for abnormal movements is important because tremors are common. Characteristics of common tremors are presented in Table 12.2. The muscles of elderly clients should also be observed for fasciculations, contractions or groups of muscle fibers that are visible, but are so localized that there is no accompanying joint movement. Fasciculations that increase on cold exposure may be a normal finding in calf muscles of elderly males. However, in elderly females or older men with increasing weakness and marked atrophy of the musculature, further testing for signs of neuromuscular disease (for example, electromyelographic studies) should be done (Burrage, 1991, p. 86).

In order to elicit latent muscle weakness caused by mild residual hemiparesis for which the client unconsciously compensates, it is important to test for drift. Drift is tested by asking the client to stand with eyes closed while holding arms straight out with palms facing each other for 20 to 30 seconds. Drift in lower extremities is tested by asking the client to sit with legs extended, eyes closed, and feet together. When minimal muscle weakness or drift is present, the involved limb will drop to a lower level and the hand will pronate or the foot will become everted.

**TABLE 12.2 Comparison of Common Types of Tremors**

| Tremor type | Oscillation characteristics | Relation to movement | Factors that accentuate tremor | Factors that suppress tremor |
|---|---|---|---|---|
| Postural (Physiologic) | fine amplitude–usually invisible to naked eye | occur with movement or in fixed position | anxiety caffeine hyperthroidism lithium tricylclics | |
| Essential (familial/senile) | larger amplitude (visible)–frequently slower than physiologic, but faster than Parkinson's | absent at rest; accentuated by voluntary tasks requiring precision | fatigue emotional factors phenothiazines halperidol | alcohol propranolol |
| Cerebellar Disease | large, irregular, slow oscillations of progressively increased amplitude as person brings limb closer to target | occur with movement; not present while limb at rest | alcohol | |
| Parkinson's Disease | slow oscillations of relaxed, supported limb | occur with limb at rest; diminish on voluntary movement | phenothiazines halperidol | sleep voluntary movement L-dopa anticholinergics |

*Note.* Developed from *Primary Care Medicine* (2nd Ed., pp. 733–735) by A. Goroll, L. May, and A. Muller, 1987. Philadelphia: J. Lippincott.

If there is any suspicion of meningitis or subarachnoid hemorrhage, tests for signs of meningeal irritation should be done. Neck stiffness due to cervical spondylosis, however, may make it difficult to evaluate the test for Brudzinski's sign (flexing the supine client's head toward the sternum while watching for resistance to the movement, pain, and hip or knee flexibility) (Carter, 1986). In this case, Kernig's sign would be more useful, since it does not require neck flexibility. Testing for Kernig's sign involves having the client supine, with leg flexed at the hip, while the lower leg is extended, and observing for resistance, pain, or inability to extend the leg (Malasanos, Barkaustas, Moss et al., 1986).

## Cerebellar Function

Testing for cerebellar function includes assessment of coordinated movement and equilibratory proprioceptive testing of posture, gait, and standing balance. In regard to coordination, the older person will usually show a decreased range of speed of fine finger movements (akinesia). Changes in handwriting are usually apparent if compared with earlier samples; it tends to become smaller and more cramped in appearance. There should be little deterioration in simpler, single tasks, such as touching the examiner's finger and the client's own nose once. However, coordinated series of movements, such as repeated finger-to-nose testing and rapid alternating movements of hands and/or feet, will show more severe deterioration. The heel-to-shin test can be done with the client sitting or supine. At least one test of coordinated movement of the upper extremities and lower extremities should be done. When one of these tests demonstrates an abnormality, additional procedures should be done to verify the problem.

In testing for posture and gait in the older person, the practitioner should observe both normal walking on a flat surface and stair climbing. Standing balance should be intact and Romberg test results negative; however, elderly persons may have some difficulty maintaining their balance during the Romberg test, perhaps due to impaired proprioception. As with any client when doing the Romberg test, the examiner should be ready to support the older client in case of severe swaying or falling when eyes are closed. To assure the older client that the examiner will not let him or her fall, the examiner's arms should encircle the client (without touching) before the request to close the eyes is made (Ryodorp, 1981). The older client's ability to stand on one leg is frequently impaired, possibly due more to proprioceptive and sensory loss than to muscle weakness or cerebellar dysfunction (Katzman & Terry, 1983). The healthy older person may have slightly increased difficulty in accomplishing tandem walking, but this ability remains basically intact (Potviu, Synduklo, Tourtellotte et al., 1980).

Careful observation of the older client while he or she is walking may reveal common age changes. The gait of a healthy older person is characterized by mild anteroflexion of the upper body, slight flexion of the arms and knees, decreased arm swing, and shortened steps with a slight widening of the distance between the feet. The velocity of gait and the stride length have been found to be sensitive indicators of gait pathology and risk of falls (Imms & Edholm, 1981).

Common neurological causes of abnormal gait in the elderly include impaired proprioception, cerebellar or vestibular system dysfunction, a central or peripheral CNS disorder, or normal pressure hydrocephalus. Physical examination findings that suggest a neurogenic gait abnormality include broad base (feet wider apart than normal), unusual lifting or dragging of leg or foot, slow ambulation, deviation of the trunk from side to side, and/or an audible sound (scraping, dragging, flopping, stamping) accompanying gait (Gambert, 1987, pp. 323–325).

Common types of abnormal gaits that may be observed in elderly clients are depicted in Figure 12.1. In Parkinson's syndrome, a propulsive gait with tiny shuffling steps and loss of associated arm movements is observed. In normal-pressure hydrocephalus, initiating the gait is difficult and step height is reduced, resulting in a shuffling gait in which the feet appear to be stuck to the floor. The client with hemiparesis will drag the affected leg or swing it forward with a circular motion. The examiner must differentiate these gait changes from those due to joint pain or stiffness.

## Deep Tendon Reflexes

Testing of deep tendon reflexes may be difficult with the older client because limb relaxation is more difficult to achieve than with the young adult. This may be due to pain and/or anxiety. It is often necessary to use reinforcement techniques to distract and relax the older adult. These include having the client concentrate on a voluntary isometric exercise (such as clenching of the fists or teeth, or pushing against something resistant) so as to achieve adequate muscle relaxation.

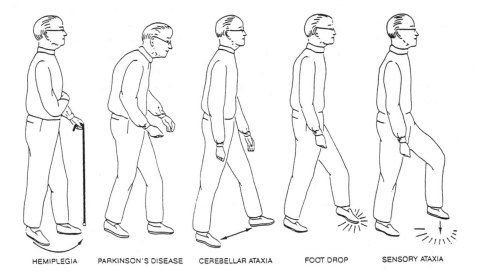

HEMIPLEGIA        PARKINSON'S DISEASE    CEREBELLAR ATAXIA        FOOT DROP        SENSORY ATAXIA

**FIGURE 12.1 Common types of abnormal gaits seen in older adults.**

From M. Schwartz, *Textbook of Physical Diagnosis: History and Examination.* 1989. Philadelphia: W.B. Saunders (p. 514). Reprinted with permission.

Severe arthritis of the knee may make the patellar reflex difficult to obtain. Locating the tendon by palpation and tapping on the examiner's finger over the tendon may be helpful. The Achilles reflex is best tested, if possible, by having the client kneel on a padded chair, with reinforcement achieved by the client clenching the chair back. An alternative method that was used to elicit the ankle jerk in 80% of elderly subjects involves having the client lie with the legs parallel while the examiner strikes his or her own fingers overlying the plantar surface of the client's dorsiflexed foot (Impallomeni, Flynn, Kenny et al., 1984). Whichever technique is used, it is important to test each reflex as soon as the instructions to relax the client and reinforce the reflex are given, since with repeated attempts, relaxation will become more difficult to achieve.

In testing the plantar reflex it is important that the feet be warm. A severe hallux valgus (bunion) or arthritis may make it difficult to judge the direction of large toe movement when attempting to elicit the plantar reflex. Decreased sensitivity due to thickening and hardening of the sole of the foot may also make the plantar response more difficult to elicit and interpret (Carotenuto & Bullock, 1980).

Reflex responses may normally be slightly increased or decreased in the older person (for example, in a range from 1+ to 3+). In advanced old age, reflexes are more likely to be decreased or absent (1+ or 0). As at any age, left and right asymmetry of reflex responses may be more significant than symmetrical differences. Results of one study of 100 aged clients without organic disease of the central nervous system indicated that upper extremity reflexes were elicited in 93%; patellar reflexes were elicited in 87%; and the Achilles reflex in 69% of the study population (Rossman, 1986). An incidence of Achilles areflexia ranging from 27% to 40% (with a larger percentage as age increases) has been reported in various studies of older people, even with the use of reinforcement techniques (Burrage, 1991). Starer and Libow contend that, with skillful technique, the ankle jerk can be elicited in most elderly.

Superficial abdominal reflexes usually disappear with age (Wolfson & Katzman, 1983). Primitive frontal release reflexes may re-emerge with aging and are sometimes elicited in otherwise normal elderly individuals; however, they may also be signs of cerebral injury or degenerative disease. The snout reflex (pursing of the lips when the upper lip is lightly tapped), the palmomental reflex (twitching of the chin when the thenar surface of the palm is scratched), and the corneomandibular reflex (lateral deviation of the mandible to the side opposite the cornea stimulated with a wisp of cotton) are the three frontal release reflexes most commonly encountered. The presence of one or two of these reflexes in a healthy elderly person is not unusual, while the presence of all three is more likely to be associated with pathologic conditions (Isakov, Sazbon, Costeff et al., 1984). A positive glabellar blink (continued reflex blinking throughout a period of 8 to 10 rapid taps on the client's frontal bone between the eyebrows) may indicate cortical or basal ganglia dysfunction. Normally the lids blink in response to the first several taps and then remain open (Jenkyn, Reeves, Warren et al., 1985).

## Sensory Function

Testing of sensory function may be difficult if there is any alteration in mental status, because it requires sustained attention to discriminate repeated stimuli. It is important to give the older client time to respond. If the client shows any signs of fatigue, hyper-distractability, or negativism, try to reschedule sensory testing for another time.

In the normal person, you would not expect to find significant decreases in perception of light touch or superficial pain; but you would expect to find increased reaction time and decreased perception of deep pain and temperature stimuli. It is important that the client's hands and feet be warm when testing vibratory sense and that it be tested on both the upper and lower extremities. Vibratory testing on the malleoli is more reliable than testing on the toes. Vibratory sense is occasionally decreased in the fingers of older adults. There is little decrease in this sensory modality in the lower extremities before age 70. Approximately 50% of older persons manifest decreased vibratory sense at the ankle, and this usually correlates with a loss of the Achilles reflex response. In addition, 15% to 30% of older persons may show a decrease or absence of position sense in the large toe (Carter, 1986). It is unclear whether these changes are normal or abnormal; therefore, spinal cord compression or disease and neuropathy need to be ruled out.

## Implications for Practice

Normal aspects of the neurological functioning of older clients should be reinforced so as to reassure the older client. The practitioner can play a significant primary prevention role with regard to the neurologic status of the older client by supporting continuance of mental and physical activity to maintain cognitive function and motor strength and agility, by improving nutritional intake patterns, and by helping the client to modify risk factors such as stress, smoking, and alcohol intake. In addition, teaching regarding appropriate use of medications that adversely affect neurological functioning may prevent falls and other types of accidents.

In the area of secondary prevention, the practitioner should recognize older clients with a high-risk profile for stroke and/or a history of TIAs, and provide counseling, teaching, and referral for medical treatment aimed at reducing the likelihood of a stroke. If decreased sensation or impaired balance are found to be present during the health assessment, the older client should be taught how to avoid injuries (for example, burns, or falls) as a result of these deficits. Older clients who require prolonged bedrest may have decreased proprioceptive sense in their feet and require assistance when beginning to ambulate.

In summary, neurological functioning is an important area in the health assessment of the older client. The data obtained can be utilized by the practitioner as a sound basis for nursing interventions directed toward promoting and maintaining the older client's health and functional abilities.

## REFERENCES

Adams, R. D., & Victor, M. (1989). *Principles of Neurology* (4th ed.) (pp. 449–456). New York: McGraw-Hill.

Besdine, R. W. (1990). Clinical evaluation of the elderly patient. In Hazzard, W. R., Andres, R., Bierman, E. L., & Blass, J. P. (Eds.), *Principles of geriatric medicine and gerontology*. New York: McGraw-Hill.

Bonikowski, F. P. (1983). Differential diagnosis of dizziness in the elderly. *Geriatrics, 38*, 89–104.

Burrage, R. L. (1991). Physical assessment: Musculoskeletal and nervous systems. In Chenitz, W. C., Stone, J. T., & Salisbury, S. A. (Eds.), *Clinical gerontological nursing: A guide to advanced practice* (pp. 82–83). Philadelphia: Saunders.

Carotenuto, R., & Bullock, J. (1980). *Physical assessment of the gerontologic client*. Philadelphia: F.A. Davis.

Carter, A. B. (1986). The neurologic aspects of aging. In Rossman, I. (Ed.), *Clinical geriatrics* (3rd ed.) (pp. 326–351). Philadelphia: J.B. Lippincott.

Gallo, J. J., Reichel, W., & Andersen, L. (1988). *Handbook of geriatric assessment* (p. 160). Gaithersburg, MD: Aspen Publishing Co.

Gambert, S. R. (1987). *Handbook of geriatrics* (p. 323). New York: Plenum Medical Book Co.

Imms, F. J., & Edholm, O. G. (1981). Studies of gait and mobility in the elderly. *Aging, 10*, 147–156.

Impallomeni, M., Flynn, M. D., Kenny, R. A. et al. (1984). The elderly and their ankle jerks. *Lancet, 1*(8378), 670–672.

Isakov, E., Sazbon, L., Costeff, H. et al. (1984). The diagnostic value of three common primitive reflexes. *European Neurology, 23*, 17–21.

Jenkyn, L. R., Reeves, A. G., Warren, T. et al. (1985). Neurologic signs in senescence. *Archives of Neurology, 42,* 1154–1157.

Joynt, R. J. (1990). Normal aging and patterns of neurologic disease. In Abrams, W. B. & Berkow, R. (Eds.), *The Merck manual of geriatrics.* Rahway, NJ: Merck, Sharp & Dohme.

Katzman, R., & Terry, R. (1983). Normal aging of the nervous system. In Katzman, R. (Ed.), *The neurology of aging* (pp. 15–50). Philadelphia: F.A. Davis.

Locke, S., & Galabarda, A. M. (1978). Neurological disorders in the elderly. In Reichel, W. (Ed.), *Clinical aspects of aging* (pp. 133–138). Baltimore: Williams & Wilkins.

Malasanos, L., Barkauskas, V., Moss, M. et al. (1986). *Health assessment* (3rd ed.). St. Louis: C. V. Mosby.

Potviu, A. R., Synduklo, K., Tourtellotte, W. E. et al. (1980). Human neurologic function and the aging process. *Journal of the American Geriatric Society, 28*(1), 1–9.

Rossman, I. (1986). *Clinical geriatrics* (3rd ed.) (p. 24). Philadelphia: J.B. Lippincott.

Rysdorp, K. (1981). Movement characteristics in the elderly. In Folmer, A .N. J. & Schouten, J. (Eds.), *Geriatrics for the practitioner.* Proceedings of a Seminar Held in Amsterdam (pp. 135–142). Princeton: Exerpta Medica.

Shaumberg, H. H., Spencer, P. S., & Ochoa, J. (1983). The aging human peripheral nervous system. In Katzman, R., & Terry, R. (Eds.), *The neurology of aging* (pp. 111–112). Philadelphia: F. A. Davis.

Starer, P. J., & Libow, S. W. (1990). History and physical examination. In W. B. Abrams & R. Berkow (Eds.), *The Merck manual of geriatrics* (p. 165). Rahway, NJ: Merck, Sharpe & Dohme.

Stone, J. T., & Chenitz, W. C. (1991). The problem of falls. In Chenitz, W. C., Stone, J. T., & Salisbury, S. A. (Eds.), *Clinical gerontological nursing: A guide to advanced practice* (pp. 304–305). Philadelphia: Saunders.

Wolfson, L. I., & Katzman, R. (1983). The neurologic consultation at age 80. In Katzman, R., & Terry, R. (Eds.), *The neurology of aging* (pp. 221–222). Philadelphia: F. A. Davis.

## SUGGESTED READINGS

Calkins, E. (Ed.). (1990). *The practice of geriatrics* (2nd ed.). Philadelphia: W.B. Saunders.

Chenitz, W. C., Stone, J. T., & Salisbury, S. A. (Eds.). (1991). *Clinical gerontological nursing: A guide to advanced practice.* Philadelphia: Saunders.

Eliopoulos, C. (1990). *Health assessment of the older adult.* Redwood City, CA: Addison-Wesley Nursing, A Division of the Benjamin/Cummings Publishing Co., Inc.

Gallo, J. J., Reichel, W., & Andersen, L. (1988). *Handbook of geriatric assessment.* Gaithersburg, MD: Aspen Publishing Co.

Gambert, S. R. (Ed.). (1987). *Handbook of geriatrics.* New York: Plenum Medical Book Co.

Hazzard, W. R., Andres, R., Bierman, E. L., & Blass, J. P. (Eds.) (1990). *Principles of geriatric medicine and gerontology* (2nd ed.). New York: McGraw-Hill.

Reichel, W. (Ed.) (1989). *Clinical aspects of aging* (3rd ed.). Baltimore: Williams & Wilkins.

Rossman, I. (Ed.) (1986). *Clinical geriatrics* (3rd ed.). Philadelphia: J.B. Lippincott.

# 13

# Assessment of Community, Home, and Nursing Home

Contrary to popular belief, it is estimated that at any one time 95% of the population over 65 are living in the community. Although nearly 30% live alone, 67% of noninstitutionalized elderly live in family settings and 18% live with their children (Staab & Lyler, 1990). The majority of older persons are able to function within their homes and communities with the help of family, friends, and a variety of support services, often despite serious physical disabilities.

Numerous surveys of the elderly indicate that their first preference is to have maximum privacy and independence in a self-owned, detached, single-family dwelling. In declining order they next prefer: to live with another person of the same age and sex; to live near or with family; and last, to live in an institution. The role that nursing and other health services should take in providing health promotion and maintenance services to the noninstitutionalized elderly is to enable them to continue to live in their preferred environment for as long as possible.

Stresses on both patients and family caregivers often result in a decision to relocate an elderly person to a more sheltered living environment. Full assessment of a patient's needs, the burden experienced by a family caregiver and options available in the community can help to avoid a forced choice made under the stress of an emergency. Many stressors experienced by the elderly, such as bereavement, retirement, decreased income, and decreased physical mobility and cognitive function, tend to isolate older people from the community. Health practitioners should become familiar with factors in the social, community, and home setting that contribute to the elderly person's health problems. Practitioners need to be cognizant of stresses on both patients and family caregivers that can be overwhelming.

There is often a discrepancy between the older person's needs, problems resulting from normal age changes or coexistent disease processes, and social–environmental factors. For example, a practitioner in a clinic who interviews an elderly client with symptoms of anorexia and nutritional deficits must consider possible client problems in procuring and preparing appetizing food as well as the possibility of age changes and disease processes that may cause these symptoms.

A practitioner working with clients who are maintaining themselves in their own homes and neighborhoods can utilize knowledge of normal age changes and common illnesses to assess whether the conditions within the home and the community are adequate to meet the needs of individual and groups of elderly clients. Some of the criteria that may be used in assessing the community and home setting include whether they provide for the following:

1. physical needs for adequate food, clothing, and shelter
2. physical and psychological safety
3. positive quality of life
4. continued social participation by older adults who wish to remain within the mainstream of social life.

This chapter will outline aspects of the community and home setting that should be of major concern to the practitioner in assessing the health status of older persons. This information may be gathered from older clients, family members, or friends, especially when the practitioner is not familiar with the client's neighborhood or is unable to make a home visit. However, the full interplay of the older client and his or her environment will be much more fully and accurately documented by data gathered directly in the home and neighborhood. Only then can the practitioner accurately determine the "fit" between the older client's needs and the home or community conditions, resources, and services.

When a problem with "fit" is identified that cannot be removed by adapting the home environment and/or securing additional support services, relocation may be necessary. Therefore, a brief overview of areas to be considered when planning for relocation is also included in this chapter. The depth and extent of community and/or home assessment that is appropriate and practical may vary with the particular purpose of the assessment and the time available to the practitioner. For example, a community health nurse working with an older population over an extended time will need to do a much more thorough community assessment than is usually feasible or necessary in planning for health care of an individual client. The assessment areas described in this chapter, however, will help the practitioner to gather maximum data during even a brief visit to the older client's home and neighborhood.

# FRAMEWORK FOR ASSESSMENT

## Person-Environment Interaction

Community and home assessment involves exploring the meaning of these environments for older people and the ways in which they are linked. In examining the mutual influences between discrete environments and older individuals, gerontologists have viewed people as proactive, and people and environments as integrated and mutually defining (Werner, Altman, & Oxley, 1985), and transacting (Lawton, 1980).

Community and home assessment involves evaluating person-environment transaction, including the characteristics of the older individual's home and community that may act either as facilitators or barriers in relation to his or her performance of basic and instrumental ADLs, cognition, and social behavior. Lawton and Nahemow's (1973) environmental press-competence model suggests that, for any given level of competence in these domains, there is a range of environmental press (or demands) within which the behavioral outcome will be favorable. In contrast, environmental demands that are too high or too low will result in maladaptive behavior and/or a negative emotional state.

The related concept of person–environment congruences (Kahana, 1982) proposes that, when there is not a good match between an individual's capabilities and the environmental press, interventions that decrease or increase environmental demands may enhance behavioral outcomes. According to Lawton and Simon's (1968) environmental hypothesis, objective environmental deficits have a greater impact on the behavior of the marginally independent user as compared to the fully able and independent individual. An environmental feature that is not a problem for most users may constitute an impenetrable barrier for an impaired elderly person.

The elderly are generally more vulnerable to environmental pressures than the young, and the extent to which their finances are inadequate, their health and functional abilities are compromised, and/or they are socially isolated will influence the degree of negative impact environmental deficits will have. On the positive side, improvements in the environmental design and quality may have a disproportionately strong positive impact on maintaining the health and functional ability of well elders and on improving the behavioral capacity of impaired older people (Lawton, 1987a).

In a further evolution of his theory, Lawton (1987a, 1987b) suggests an environmental proactivity hypotheses which complements his environmental docility hypothesis: As competence increases, the environment becomes a potential source of increasing diversity in the person's ability to satisfy needs; the person's behavioral space can then be richer and more demanding, as well as potentially more satisfying. The environmental docility and proactivity hypotheses represent a basic dialectic in regard to creating ideal environments of older persons— the dialectic of providing support versus promoting autonomy. While decline and deprivation demand support, the human spirit demands autonomy. The challenge is to create adequately, but not overly protective environments (wherein the press level is consistent with competencies) that still allow the exercise of individual autonomy.

## COMMUNITY ASSESSMENT

### Overall Features

A summary of the components of a community assessment is presented in Table 13.1. In trying to gain a general impression of the community, the practitioner needs to learn something of the past and recent history of the neighborhood. This should include whether the neighborhood is growing or contracting, stable or changing; whether it seems to be attractive and to offer a positive quality of life; and whether it is perceived by elderly residents as a pleasant and secure place to live. The climate is of concern because extremes in climatic conditions pose health problems for older people. A very cold climate increases thermoregulatory and mobility problems as well as joint, cardiovascular, and respiratory symptoms. Very warm and humid conditions also increase the severity of cardiac and respiratory problems. A mild, warm, dry climate is most beneficial to the elderly. The location of the community in a rural, suburban, or urban area, and whether the neighborhood is in the center or on the periphery of the town are also significant.

**TABLE 13.1 Community Assessment Guide**

*Overall features*

| Climate | Roadways | Noise level |
|---|---|---|
| Location | Open space | Economic state |
| Topography | Distribution of buildings | Community planning |

*Population characteristics*

| Overall age, sex, ethnic distribution | Ethnic/socioeconomic characteristics of elderly |
|---|---|
| Proportion of elderly in population | Intergenerational relations |

*Service facilities*

| *Shopping/basic services* | *Educational* |
|---|---|
| Food, drug, clothing stores | Public library |
| Dry cleaners | Adult education programs |
| Shoe repair | |
| Restaurants | |
| Banks | |
| Post office | |

| *Health care* | *Social/recreational* |
|---|---|
| Ambulance service | Places of worship |
| Clinics | Outdoor parks |
| Hospitals | Indoor facilities: |
| Physicians | The "Y" |
| Dentists | Cinemas |
| Home care services | Bowling |
| Pharmacists | Private clubs |
| Folk healers | |

| *Social services* | *Transportation* |
|---|---|
| Social security office | Private cars |
| Welfare office | Taxis |
| Senior citizens' programs: | Subways and/or buses |
| Senior centers, clubs, nutrition programs, outreach services | |

*Environmental/safety conditions*

| Pavement/curbs | Air quality | Police department (crime rate) |
|---|---|---|
| Crosswalks | Sanitation services | |
| Street lighting | Unleashed animals | Fire department (fire, arson rate) |

*Source:* Adapted from *Community Assessment Guide*, Lehman College Department of Nursing, CUNY, Bronx, New York, 1975.

Noting the topography of the neighborhood is relevant, since a hilly terrain puts additional stress on the diminished cardiovascular and respiratory reserves of older people. The pattern and type of roadways are of concern in regard to accessibility and ease of transportation. Pedestrian safety, air quality, and environmental noise are major concerns for mobile senior citizens with sensory deficits and slowed reaction times. The amount of open space as compared with the number and distribution of buildings is significant. In downtown areas natural elements, such as parks, gardens, and landscaped areas, may be of particular importance because the elderly are more accustomed to them than to modern concrete and steel environments and because the elderly have more leisure time to enjoy them (Evans, Brennan, Skorpanich, & Held, 1984).

The location of light or heavy industry and the placement of local shops and businesses may have an important impact on the quality of life and ease of meeting basic needs. The types, duration, and intensity of environmental sounds can be assessed in relation to their impact on the older adult who has decreased ability to hear high-pitched sounds and to discriminate background sounds that are ordinarily important in alerting cues to hazards. The observed state of the community as thriving or deteriorating gives evidence of its economic state. Evidence of community planning for the elderly population, such as housing and services, should be noted. Accessibility to and participation in the political process by older members of the community should be evaluated.

## Population Characteristics

In recent decades the movement of the urban younger population to suburban areas and the concentration of the older age group in the inner cities have been well-documented. Many urban elderly do not wish to leave familiar surroundings or they are "locked in" by poverty. Such individuals may become isolated in neighborhoods undergoing rapid change, especially if most of their friends have moved away or died. However, a familiar environment, consisting of persons of all ages, and neighbors who can assist when needed, may be deemed more beneficial by some older individuals than living in improved but age-segregated housing that reinforces the older person's "end of the road" perspective.

Census tract information, available from appropriate city agencies or public libraries, can indicate the past and present age distribution within neighborhoods. Reviewing this information, observing the community, and asking questions of residents will provide information about the age, sex, socioeconomic status, and ethnic distribution of the population. As previously noted, rapid population changes can have an isolating effect on older citizens. The proportion of elderly in the community affects the local tax base, general employment level, and relative purchasing power and it may influence intergenerational conflicts. If the elderly are of a different ethnic group from the younger people or new arrivals, this may cause language and other communication barriers. It is important to determine how elderly and younger residents view each other, and whether the older person feels secure and respected within the neighborhood. This perception greatly influences the older person's mental/emotional status, physical well-being, and social activity patterns. The practitioner should attempt to ascertain whether most of the elderly population in the community are living alone, with extended families, or in segregated senior citizen housing, and whether there is a "hidden" population of homebound elderly in need of outreach services.

## Service Facilities

Adequate housing is not sufficient for meeting the social and health needs of the elderly. Many older people require additional special services.

The elderly may have limited energy, mobility, and money for travel. It is very important to identify the adequacy of shopping and service facilities for such basic necessities as food, clothing, drugs, dry cleaning, shoe repair, banking, and post office. Stores should be observed for such factors as cleanliness, wide and unobstructed aisles, and adequate lighting. Large print pricing labels for comparison shopping should be noted, as well as whether prices are reasonable, food stamps are accepted, senior citizen discounts offered, and home delivery available (for example, of food or medicines). Whether the post office offers an "Early Alert" service and whether banks provide direct deposit service for social security and pension checks, as well as whether these services are used by older people, can also be identified. The availability of clean, reasonably priced restaurants, with menus appropriate to the nutritional needs of senior citizens, may be significant for older clients who prefer eating out.

The presence and location of health care services including ambulance service, ambulatory and inpatient facilities, and practitioners of medicine and dentistry, should be noted, as well as agencies that provide home care services such as skilled nursing, physical therapy, and home health aides. The quality of care provided, and whether these health care providers accept Medicare and/or Medicaid payments, should be ascertained. The availability of reputable pharmacists who offer reasonably priced generic and brand name prescriptions and who can give sound advice about over-the-counter drugs is also important. Reading local newspapers and observing storefronts can provide information regarding folk healers used by some ethnic groups.

It is important to note the location of official social service agencies, such as the nearest social security and welfare offices. The location of such social service programs for the elderly as day care, nutrition programs, or senior citizen clubs, should also be identified. Many of these programs provide additional services, such as transportation, health screening, exercise programs, discussion groups, and personal or legal counseling. The practitioner will also want to ascertain the availability of outreach services to the homebound elderly, including "Meals on Wheels," homemaker services, friendly visitors, telephone reassurance service, and respite care services for live-in caretakers—both in the home or in local nursing homes.

The public library may provide resources for both practical and leisure pursuits of the elderly. Adult education programs may be offered by local high schools and colleges. They should be investigated as to the appropriateness of topics and fees charged to senior citizens.

The location and denomination of places of worship is important to note, especially if the elderly residents in the community find strength and important social relationships in the continuing practice of their religion. Outdoor recreation areas, where the elderly may safely walk or sit in good weather, as well as appropriate public indoor recreational facilities, such as the YMCA, cinemas, bowling, and billiards, should be noted. Private neighborhood ethnic, social, or political clubs may provide meeting places to chat and play cards with old friends.

In assessing available modes of transportation it is important to note whether most of the frequently used shopping and services facilities can be reached by foot or if they require some type of transportation. If the older person does not drive or have family members available to meet transportation needs, the availability of public transportation should be ascertained. It is especially important to note if the older person has the physical abilities required to use the available modes of public transportation—taxi, bus, or subway. For example, stairs, sliding doors, and crowded conditions require a level of alertness, reaction time, vision, hearing, and physical mobility that some elderly persons may not possess. Because of the financial pressures that older persons on fixed incomes may experience, the cost of available transportation should be noted, as well as whether there are special fares for senior citizens. The location of stops, whether there are covered waiting areas with seats, and frequency of scheduling may also be important factors in the older person's ability to use available public transportation.

## Environmental/Safety Conditions

The sensory and mobility deficits prevalent in the older age group greatly increase the hazards of falling and other accidents. Therefore, it is important to observe areas of potential hazard in the community. The pavement of streets and sidewalks should provide an even walking surface, free of holes, unexpected bumps, or litter. It is important to note whether the curbs are even and provide color contrast for visibility and if the street lighting is adequate and uniform. The crosswalks at busy intersections should be well marked, with crossing light signals that are timed to allow for the slower reaction time and movement patterns of older persons. In colder climates, snow and ice removal services are important, since hazardous walking conditions will either socially isolate elderly persons or result in the increased incidence of accidental falls.

The air quality in the community has a special impact on older people with respiratory problems. A visit to the neighborhood can provide a gross estimate of any air pollution problems. The local environmental protection agency may be able to provide more specific information concerning the severity of the pollution and any related risks to health. Large numbers of unleashed animals in the neighborhood may cause additional problems for elderly residents.

Because of the increasing crime rate in many communities, the elderly are frequently victims of crime, both within and outside their homes. The availability and visibility of the police department in the neighborhood is very important. Statistics concerning the incidence rate for specific crimes to which the elderly are prey, such as burglary, mugging, and rape, may be obtained from the local police department, as well as information about special education or protective services offered to senior citizens. The location of police call boxes and fire alarm boxes should be noted. The local fire department can provide data concerning the fire and arson incidence rate in the area and its implications for elderly residents. The availability of "Neighborhood Watch" or "Senior Check Station" programs is also important.

# HOME ASSESSMENT

## Overall Features

The concept of "home" is significant for many older persons because it is part of their identity. Home is that place where things are familiar and unchanging and where people maintain some sense of autonomy and control. The majority of older people in the United States own their own homes and most view communal living as representing a loss of freedom and dignity. Nearly 80% of elderly respondents in a recent survey reported living situation preferences identical to their present arrangements (Wister, 1989). Although the majority of older individuals may wish to "age in place," some elders may not feel really at home in their living conditions. Keeping older people in their homes cannot be made a universal goal. Remaining in the home setting is beneficial only when that is where the older client wishes to live and when the living conditions are adequate and can be maintained with selected interventions.

Housing for the elderly should optimally do the following: (1) provide good shelter within the individual's financial capability; and (2) promote physical and mental well-being by providing opportunities for socialization and health maintenance while permitting privacy, independence, and continuation of one's lifestyle. It should be kept in mind that the behavioral norms of the social environment of older persons will vary according to the age heterogeneity or homogeneity of their milieu; the age differences in a heterogenous environment require much more role flexibility in regard to a wider range of experiences and demands than a milieu with a high concentration of elderly (Bernardin-Haldeman, 1988).

An increasing variety of retirement housing in the community provides alternatives to remaining in the residence where the middle adult years have been spent. Types of housing for the elderly include government-subsidized apartment houses, rental or cooperative apartments, congregate housing, retirement villages, trailer parks, residence clubs, and converted hotels. There are increasing numbers of multi-step housing complexes for the elderly, with levels ranging from independent living to board and care, to assisted living, to skilled nursing facility (Continuing Care Retirement Communities).

It would be helpful for the practitioner to know the characteristics, policies, costs, and services offered in order to assess the advantages and disadvantages of each type of senior citizen housing in the area. For example, some facilities may cost more than many elderly can afford; some may be poorly situated and isolated from the mainstream of life and services, and others may be located in high crime rate areas; some may foster more togetherness than an older individual can tolerate, or require sharing of room or bath with strangers.

Older persons tend to appraise their present residential situations more positively than outsiders do (Golant, 1986). And, because the elderly often have a decreased capacity for changing or manipulating their environment, living conditions may have more influence on their behavior than on that of younger counterparts. Research indicates that older people are more apt to engage in psychological adaptation to their environment than to change their physical or social environment; for example, they may accept more inconveniences and decrease their expectations concerning what constitutes adequate living conditions (Wister, 1989). An individual's sense of personal space is closely related to his or her sense of self and its extent usually decreases with aging. But no matter how limited its extent, an older individual's personal space should be entered only on invitation, and with evidence of respect for his or her privacy and personal integrity.

The home assessment can be done during even a brief interview and observation of the home when the practitioner has an organized framework for data collection. A summary of the components for the home assessment is presented in Table 13.2.

The practitioner should begin the home visit by ascertaining how long the older person has lived in this setting and by eliciting the person's perceptions concerning how satisfactory it is in meeting his or her needs. Observation of and discussion about valued personal objects that are displayed in the home provide unique and important windows into the person's past and present experiences, lifestyle, hobbies or occupation, and interpersonal relationships.

A baseline functional assessment can be accomplished during the home visit, including use of standard ADL, IADL, depression, and mini-

**TABLE 13.2 Home Assessment Guide**

*Roles and relationships*

| | |
|---|---|
| Quality of relationships within the home | Responsibility for money management, household tasks |
| Available support systems outside the home | Pets |

*Comfort and convenience*

| | |
|---|---|
| Home maintenance costs | Decor |
| Overall size of living quarters | Heating and ventilation |
| Spatial arrangements | |

*Safety*

| | |
|---|---|
| Floors | Particular rooms |
| Stairways |   Bathroom |
| Electrical wiring and appliances |   Kitchen |
| Exposed pipes or radiators |   Bedroom |
| Lighting | Door and window locks |
| Telephone | Smoke and fire detectors |
| | Emergency plan |
| | Safekeeping of valuables |
| | Medications |

mental status scales (see Chapter 4 & 11). The items on these questionnaires and rating scales can be integrated throughout the visit to make them less threatening. It is important to not just ask about, but have the older client demonstrate, safe functioning in the home setting (for example, in regard to ability to use the stove, microwave, phone, etc.).

## Roles and Relationships

The quality of interpersonal relationships within the home, with family members, and with neighbors, should be noted. When discussing the distribution of tasks, it is important to identify who is responsible for money management and other household maintenance tasks such as shopping, cooking, dishwashing, light and heavy cleaning, laundry, and yard work. The older person should continue to perform customary self-maintaining tasks such as dressing, bathing, and usual household tasks (if this is feasible). If a husband, after his retirement, unilaterally takes over the shopping and cooking rather than developing other new roles, this may deprive his wife of one of her most satisfying life roles. Other family members may also create unnecessary dependency and unhappiness by assuming tasks that aged members are still capable of performing for themselves. Here, again, an assessment of older individuals in their home environment will be most helpful in making judgments about the delicate balance of their independence and dependency roles.

The presence of pets in the home can also provide evidence of a fulfilling relationship, but it should also be ascertained whether the pets can be cared for properly. Dogs and cats are generally the most preferred pets. A dog can be a protection as well as a support for mental/emotional well-being. The need for exercise and cost of feeding and grooming are key factors in selecting a suitable pet. Birds or fish may also be appropriate pets.

The surveillance zone, defined as the external space within the visual field of one's home, assumes increasing significance as people grow older and spend more time at home. This zone mediates between the personal space of home and the more remote community environment beyond the visual field, thereby providing an important source of ongoing environmental participation and a sense of identity, especially for the homebound elder. It represents an arena for watching and being watched, for a visual recirpocity that facilitates the emergence and maintenance of practical and social support from neighbors. A home visit provides the practitioner with an opportunity to assess the older person's use of his or her surveillance zone, including which windows are used and the arrangement of furniture, which facilitates monitoring of the space around the home and a sense of vicarious participation in the events which occur there. In addition, the practitioner can explore information about signal systems shared with neighbors within the surveillance zone for monitoring each other's well-being and giving or receiving help during crisis situations (Rowles, 1984).

## Comfort and Convenience

The cost of living in the home (rent, taxes, utilities, and maintenance expenses) should be reasonable for the standard of living, within the limits of the older person's income. The overall size of the living quarters may be much larger than needed if older persons are still in their pre-retirement homes. If they have moved all of their furnishings into a small apartment, they may feel cramped. The arrangement of the rooms and position of the stairs should be noted in terms of convenience for accomplishing activities of daily living. The practitioner may note that the frail older individual has arranged a "control center" (Saperstein, Lawton, Moleski, & Sharp, 1984), around his or her favorite chair from which the phone, TV or radio controls, etcetera can be reached and neighborhood activities monitored.

The attractiveness of the decor (with use of warm colors and contrasting color schemes to help visual discrimination) and sturdy, supportive, well-placed furniture can do much to add to the quality of life. Although the presence of some clutter may have a therapeutic value for the elderly in providing a sense of closeness and spatial orientation, there must be enough room for ease and safety of movement. Placement of clocks and calendars in strategic locations can assist in the maintenance of time orientation. A television set and/or radio can aid both time and social orientation.

The heating and ventilation should provide for fresh air in a comfortable temperature range (ideally 70 to 75 degrees Fahrenheit, because older people have a decreased tolerance for temperature extremes). This is especially important to emphasize because of the current advocacy of lowered thermostats. Because heating the home is expensive, elderly people on fixed incomes may be forced to cut back on their heat in order to save money for food and other necessities. In winter, limiting ventilation may be an attempt to conserve heat but may result in poor air quality.

## Safety Factors

Accidents constitute the sixth leading cause of death in people over age 75 (Kay & Tideiksaar, 1990). The majority of accidents in the older population occur in the home. Falls are responsible for more of these home accidents than fires, burns, or poisoning. The elderly are at increased risk for home accidents because of multiple normal age changes and disease-related alterations in functioning. An unsteady gait may result from a number of factors including: decreased muscle strength, coordination, and balance; dizziness resulting from decreased cerebral blood flow; or medication side effects. The older person's slowed reaction time and decreased vision, hearing, and pain sensation also increase the risk of accidents; therefore, careful identification of actual or potential safety hazards should be a high priority in the home assessment. Carrying out safety measures does not necessarily require making costly structural changes. In suggesting needed changes, the practitioner can emphasize that the older person can definitely exert some control over safety in the home.

Walkways both within and outside the home should be uncluttered. Telephones, electrical cords, and hoses should not intrude into or across walkways. Additional shelving, better use of storage space, and/or eliminating clutter may be necessary to remove hazardous obstructions. Use of contrasting colors will help older people to pinpoint where the wall meets the floor or the corners of a room. Floors should have even nonskid surfaces. Avoidance of slippery surfaces in the bathroom is especially critical, since they are the cause of over 70% of all bathroom accidents (Harootyan, 1988). Wall-to-wall carpeting or large area rugs should be well-anchored, and any small rugs should have a nonskid rubber backing. Only nonskid waxes should be used on uncarpeted surfaces. Corrugated or crepe-soled shoes may also help to prevent falls on uncarpeted floors. It is advisable that the older person wear firm supportive footwear rather than soft slippers.

Because a significant proportion of falls occur on stairs, it is particularly important to inspect the condition of both indoor and outdoor stairways. The height of the steps should be uniform and the treads should be even and covered with a nonskid surface. Research indicates that stairs with 7-inch risers and an 11-inch tread depth (as required by public building codes) significantly reduce the risk of falling (Harootyan, 1988). If the client has significant visual problems, it may be helpful to mark the stair edges with a bright contrasting color. Adequate lighting of the whole stairway is also very important. Handrails should be present, easy to grasp, and placed securely. In most homes, handrails are too low for maximum safety, forcing elders with impaired balance and agility to lean foward to use the handrail. This is especially dangerous when descending the stairs (Harootyan, 1988). If the stairway is wide enough, it is helpful to have handrails on both sides so that the individual can grasp a railing with his or her dominant hand when going either up or down stairs. High or uneven thresholds at doorways may also be a mobility hazard. If the older person lives in an apartment building with an elevator, the client's level of comfort in using the elevator, as well as its ease of operation, lighting, and maintenance, can be assessed.

Electrical appliances and switches should be observed for convenience of switch locations and the condition of appliances, electrical cords, and plugs. Room space heaters, heating pads, and electrical blankets or mattress pads can be particular sources of thermal-electrical hazards for the elderly. For greater safety, older clients can be counseled to use their electric blanket or mattress pad before bedtime to warm up their bed and then to turn it off and use a comforter when they get in bed. In assessing the heating system, any exposed hot radiators or pipes should be noted. Proper maintenance and functioning of a gas furnace is important because of the risk of carbon monoxide poisoning. It should be checked annually by the utility company. The use of inappropriate sources of heat, such as indoor use of charcoal heaters, is very dangerous.

Both the natural and artificial lighting in the home should optimally provide an even general illumination of rooms and hallways via diffuse lighting from many directions. Direct supplementary lighting of the central visual field is necessary for tasks such as reading, sewing, and food preparation. There should not be an extreme contrast in the intensity of the lighting. The presence of glare reduces visual efficiency and produces eye fatigue and pain in the elderly. Therefore, light sources should be shielded from direct view and kept above the normal vision line. The older person will find it helpful to turn his or her head when switching on a bright light. Polished and glossy surfaces, such as chrome and shiny desktops or tabletops, should be eliminated, and non-glossy, light-colored matte furniture finishes used. Because of reduced dark and light adaptation and glare tolerance, special care must be taken when older people go from very bright to very dark areas.

The presence and location of a telephone is important in maintaining safety and social contact. Studies have shown that having a telephone may contribute to a longer life, since elderly persons without telephones have evidenced a significantly higher mortality rate. It should be noted whether the phone has a lighted or enlarged dial for ease of use at night or for people with visual impairment. Special phones are also available for the hard-of-hearing. The phone should be easy to reach during the day and night. Its location can be crucial. For example, if an older person is unusually fearful, it may be helpful to consider installation of an extension phone. Cellular phones, along with tissues and other necessities, may be carried in an apron which is worn or attached to a walker. Emergency numbers, including those of the nearest relative, neighbor, primary health care provider, police and fire departments, and ambulance service, should be clearly written and posted beside the telephone. It is advisable to place a "911" sticker directly on the telephone itself.

Certain rooms require more particular observation for the presence of safety hazards. In the bathroom the size of the doorways and the space around the toilet can be especially important if the client uses a walker or wheelchair. The height of the toilet is significant if the older client has decreased strength or range of motion in the lower extremities. If the seat is low, a built-up seat and/or handrails beside the toilet may be particularly helpful. Safety in the use of the tub or shower is also greatly enhanced by the presence of sturdy handrails nailed into the studs and by skid-proof mats. A stable seat with shower head extension may be helpful if the older person is not able to lower and raise himself fully in the tub or to remain standing safely in the shower. Electrical outlets should be at a safe distance from the tub and there should be ground fault interrupts in both bathroom and kitchen outlets. Slippery surfaces in the bathroom (for example, ceramic tile floors) should be minimized since they become even more slippery when wet. As in the kitchen, wall-to-wall carpeting is the safest floor surface. Area rugs should have a full size sheet rubber backing (Harootyan, 1988).

In the kitchen the stove is a major concern. Inadequate cooking facilities, such as a single-burner stove, may contribute to poor eating habits and malnutrition. The stove should be free of grease and flammable objects, and the older person should not cook while wearing long sleeves or loose night clothes. Controls should be easily accessible and readable. Electricity is the safest heat source for cooking. Because of decreased olfactory sense in the older person, a fatal gas leak may not be easily detected. There should be a pilot light on a gas stove; if there is none, safety in the use of matches and precautions to prevent gas leakage should be explored. A small fire extinguisher or container of baking soda should be kept close to the stove. Simple microwaves, with only an on–off switch, can be substituted if the client is unable to use a stove safely.

There should be adequate cold and hot (but not scalding) water for drinking, cooking, cleaning, and bathing. The pre-set temperature on the hot water heater should be set no higher than 120°F. There should be freely draining sinks and a drain trap is advisable to prevent loss of rings or other valuables down the drain.

Observation of current food supplies should corroborate the older client's nutritional history. The refrigerator should be functional and food properly labeled and stored, and not outdated or spoiled. The kitchen work areas should be well-lighted and counters should provide adequate work surfaces at a comfortable height. Storage cabinets should be easy to reach, without the need for stooping or stretching. If a step-stool is used, it should be sturdy and provide a broad base of support. The system for trash and garbage removal, general cleanliness, and the presence of any household pests should be noted. Older people with decreased vision may not see well enough to be aware of dirt accumulation or roach or ant infestation. Because the kitchen floor may get wet and then be particularly slippery, it is important that spills be wiped up immediately and that the floor have a nonskid finish. Wall-to-wall kitchen carpeting provides the safest floor surface.

In the bedroom it is important to check the height and firmness of the mattress in relation to the older client's height, mobility problems, and back pain. A lamp and flashlight, as well as a phone, should be within easy reach beside the bed, and it is advisable to have night lights well placed to illuminate the route to the bathroom. Use of a urinal or bedside commode may decrease likelihood of falling on the way to the bathroom at night.

Another safety and security measure to include in the assessment is the type and condition of door and window locks. Exterior doors should have deadbolt locks which cannot be easily forced open by an intruder (for example, with a credit card). If windows are barred, there should be a quick release mechanism to allow rapid exit in an emergency. There should be a well-maintained smoke or fire detection system, including a detector placed near the kitchen (but not too near the stove). The older person should have developed a plan for meeting emergencies (alternate exits for escape in case of fire). If the older person or family members smoke, evidence of unsafe smoking habits should be noted.

It is important to determine how valuables have been secured. Some older people keep their cash or other valuables in their mattresses, rather than placing them in the bank for safekeeping. It should also be ascertained whether weapons are kept in the home and whether it is advisable that the gun(s) and/or ammunition should be removed or at least locked up.

It is essential for the practitioner to investigate where and how medications (both prescription and over-the-counter) are stored and if they are correctly labeled. In addition, stores of alcoholic beverages (if any) should be checked. Medications should not be used beyond their expiration date. Older people may keep old medications, even those prescribed for another family member, and use them inappropriately or when they are no longer effective. Multiple medications may be combined in one bottle so that the labeling is incorrect. These practices increase the possibility of medication errors and untoward reactions. Any problem noted in regard to the handling of medications, nutritional supplements, or folk remedies (for example, herbal preparations) requires prompt intervention. Table 13.3 presents a Safety Interview Guide and Checklist that can be used in doing a focused assessment of physical, psychosocial, and lifestyle-related safety factors in frail elder's home environment.

## GUIDELINES FOR ASSISTING ELDERS AND THEIR FAMILIES TO SELECT A NURSING HOME

Although it is true that at any one time only 5% of the nation's elderly are living in institutions, one out of four will spend time in a nursing home at some point in their later years (Kemper & Murtaugh, 1991). The longer people live, the greater the likelihood that they will develop disabling conditions that require temporary or continuous protective or skilled care. If finances are adequate, and needed services available, this care can be provided in the community. When this is not the case, or when nursing home placement is preferred, elders and their families who have investigated nursing homes in advance will be better prepared to make a sound choice that takes into account the older person's attitudes and preferences. Rushed decisions and placements in crisis situations not only limit the options, but also do not allow time for elders and their families to prepare themselves emotionally for this important life transition (Silverstone & Hyman, 1982).

When assessment suggests the likelihood of future institutional care the practitioner can play a key role in assisting the older individual and/or family members to explore the possibilities ahead of time. This section describes steps to follow in selecting a nursing home and criteria for evaluating available institutional settings. The practitioner can share this information with elders and their families to increase the likelihood of successful placement when the need arises. It must be remembered that an essential ingredient in all of the planning is the step-by-step involvement of the potential nursing home resident in what may be one of his or her last major life decisions. Even if the older person is not able to visit the possible homes, he or she may be able to comprehend written information and verbal reports about them and express preferences and priorities during the decision-making process (Slack, 1986).

## TABLE 13.3 Home Safety Interview Guide and Checklist

This tool is designed for use in the elderly client's home or in primary care office or clinic settings to facilitate the identification of safety risk factors and the prevention of injuries among elderly clients through appropriate interventions to reduce these risk factors. This interview guide and checklist comprise a cost-effective tool that can be used by professional or para-professional personnel to guide their focused assessment of safety factors/hazards in the elderly client's home environment and/or lifestyle.

The information is ideally obtained in the client's home but, when this is not possible, may alternatively be gathered during elderly clients' visits to busy primary care offices or clinics. The information can then be used as a basis for discussion with the older client, as well as his or her caregiver(s) and family members, of the safety risks identified and recommendations for eliminating or, at least, reducing them. The completed Home Safety Interview Guide and Checklist can be kept in the client's health record along with recommendations for reducing the identified safety risks; it can later be used to evaluate whether the recommended preventive actions have, indeed, been implemented.

Name_____

Date_____                    Interviewer_____

Caregiver—Self

other (name, relationship, phone number)
How helpful is caregiver?
Does caregiver have help? (who, when?)
Is caregiver stressed? Fatigued?
Does caregiver have health problems?

Patient— What health problems do you have?
What medicines do you take? (Ask patient to bring all medicines
to office.)
Where are your medicines kept?
Do you use a medicine box or a calendar?
Do you drink beer, wine or hard liquor? How much?
Do you smoke? How much?
Do you have memory loss?
Have you ever gotten lost outside of your home?
Do you see or hear things other people do not see or hear?
Exercise—What type? How often?
Finances—Source? Adequate to meet your needs?
Vision—Adequate? Impared? Glasses?
         Date of last exam?
Hearing—Adequate? Impaired?
         Do you wear a hearing aid?
Mobility— Have you fallen within the last year?
         Are you afraid of falling?
         Do you ever use a cane or walker?
         Can you go up and down the stairs easily?
         Do you drive? Is your license current?
Nutrition—Who prepares meals?
         Appetite
         Weight loss—Stable, loss, gain

*(continued)*

**TABLE 13.3** (*continued*)

|  | Yes | No | Comments |
|---|---|---|---|
| Swimming pool |  |  |  |
| Steps |  |  |  |
| Railings |  |  |  |
| Smoke alarm |  |  |  |
| Barred windows—(quick release) |  |  |  |
| Electric blanket/mattress pad |  |  |  |
| Electric space heater |  |  |  |
| Night lights |  |  |  |
| Gas furnace— (should be checked yearly by utility company) |  |  |  |
| Scatter rugs |  |  |  |
| Grab rail in tub or shower |  |  |  |
| Does toilet seat need to be elevated? |  |  |  |
| Are grab rails needed? |  |  |  |
| Are walkways cluttered? |  |  |  |
| Do extension or phone cords intrude? |  |  |  |
| Can patient summon help in an emergency? |  |  |  |
| Does patient know emergency phone number (911)? |  |  |  |
| Are weapons kept in the home? |  |  |  |
| Are guns loaded? Locked? |  |  |  |
| Do doors have dead bolts? |  |  |  |
| What is preset temperature on water heater? |  |  |  |
| Does a family member, friend or neighbor have a key to your house? |  |  |  |
| Can you see who is at the front door before you open the door? |  |  |  |
| Are walkways in front of home even? |  |  |  |
| Do hoses or vegetation block walkways? |  |  |  |

*Source:* SOCARE (Seniors Only Care) Clinic, University of California San Diego Medical Center, 225 Dickinson St., San Diego, CA 92013. Used with permission.

## Step One: Financial Considerations

The first step in choosing a nursing home is understanding how money determines the individual's options. Private nursing home care is very expensive; however, the older person who can pay for nursing home care for at least some initial period of time has a wider range of options. Many nursing homes do not accept individuals who must be admitted on Medicaid. Therefore, the client's eligibility for Medicare and Medicaid may be an important initial consideration.

Medicare coverage is limited to post-hospital care for up to 100 days in an approved nursing facility for specified "treatable" conditions that require skilled nursing services on a daily basis; the average length of coverage is 2 weeks and only a small percentage of nursing home residents qualify. Because of the numerous regulations associated with it, many nursing homes do not seek Medicare certification. In contrast, Medicaid covers the cost of long-term care for eligible low-income persons in licensed nursing homes for as long as their condition merits it. Veteran's benefits may entitle certain older individuals to residence in a veteran's home or in other types of nursing homes that have arrangements with the Veteran's Administration.

Individuals with limited resources should be referred to their local Social Security office, Department of Social Services (Welfare) office, Area Agency on Aging, and/or Medicaid office for assistance in applying for Medicaid. Although federal regulations mandate that Medicaid payments are based on need, each state sets its own eligibility requirements. To establish financial need, the Medicaid application must usually provide copies of recent bank statements, a copy of the social secruity award letter or most recent social security check, proof of the cash value of any life insurance policies, bonds, or other liquefiable assets, and proof of income amounts from any other sources. To the extent that the total value of assets exceeds the state mandated limit, the person will have to "spend down" before becoming eligible for Medicaid to pick up their nursing home costs.

Under today's Medicaid regulations, adult children are no longer held financially accountable for their parents' nursing home bills. However, older individuals who are contemplating the need for nursing home placement, and/or their families, may need guidance from a lawyer concerning what can be done legally in the particular state to prevent impoverishment of the "healthy" spouse who will continue to live in the community, while allowing the nursing home resident to be eligible for Medicaid; for example, splitting of the couple's assets. The Medicaid worker who handles the application can also be consulted about whether a maintenance allowance for spouse and/or dependents living at home can be negotiated and/or a grace period granted during which a portion of the nursing home resident's monthly income can be used to maintain his or her previous dwelling (to allow the possibility of re-entrance into the community should health status improve or the placement prove unsatisfactory).

## Step Two: Identifying the Kinds of Care Available

All nursing home facilities are not alike; they may offer one or more of the levels of care recognized in the federal laws that regulate Medicare and Medicaid. Some nursing facilities provide 24-hour-a-day supervision and treatment by a registered nurse (RN); they are appropriate for persons who need continuous nursing supervision in addition to other services; for example, for short-term rehabilitation periods following illness or surgery, or for chronic conditions that require continuous skilled nursing interventions and supervision. In contrast, other facilities, previously known as intermediate care facilities (ICFs), are suitable for persons who are not capable of independent living, but who require only limited nursing services. The emphasis in these facilities is on personal care and socialization. Another type of facility is the board and care, or retirement home (Residential Facilities for the Elderly, or RFEs), which provide nonmedical care and supervision that may include personal care services (for example, bathing, grooming, taking self-administered medication), and help with activities of daily living.

Older individuals and their families should be counseled not to select a facility that provides more care than he or she needs because this involves more expense and may encourage dependence on the part of the resident. However, if the person is likely to need more care in the future, a facility that offers multiple levels of care would be preferable. The availability of different types of care in the same setting would enable the older person to be shifted smoothly from one level to another when needed, which is much less traumatic to the resident and family than a move to another institution.

The practitioner can provide guidance regarding the type(s) of care that will be needed and/or refer the older person and family to their physician, a qualified medical social worker, or the nursing home admission team for a more specific needs assessment. Careful delineation of the care likely to be required can prevent inappropriate placement followed by the trauma of transfer to a different level of care or even back to the community.

## Step Three: Identifying and Narrowing the Options

Once the level of care required and the financial resources available to provide that care have been determined, it is important that the interested parties become informed about nursing homes in the area. Agencies such as the county Area Agency on Aging, or the Senior Information and Referral Office, the Nursing Home Ombudsman, or the local state medical assistance (Medicaid) office are good places to start. All of these organizations should have a list of area nursing homes and their specifications. It is also recommended that the older person and/ or family members talk with nurses, physicians, social workers, and clergy who are knowledgeable about area nursing homes, as well as with friends who work in or have family members living in them. These people can provide important experience-based information about the track record of particular nursing homes.

It may be essential to determine at the outset whether the nursing homes being considered are approved for reimbursement under Medicare and Medicaid and the availability of "Medicaid beds." Nursing homes often strictly limit the number of beds set aside for individuals covered by Medicaid and have long waiting lists for these beds. They may more readily admit private pay residents on short notice and they often allow them to remain, even after their resources are depleted and they become eligible for Medicaid. Residents accepted by a nursing home will receive comparable care regardless of whether they are private pay, Medicare, or Medicaid. It may be more difficult, however, to find an available bed for an individual who qualifies for Medicaid prior to admission. It may be necessary to apply at a number of homes and be assertive about calling back if the older person has been placed on a waiting list.

## Step Four: Comparing Available Facilities to Determine the Best Match

The next step is to try to match the preferences of the older person with the available options. Major factors to be considered in relation to each nursing home are: ownership or management, size, location, nursing care and other services offered, and convenience for the individual's family members, friends, and physician.

In regard to ownership and management, nursing homes are either "nonprofit" or "for profit" (proprietary). Nonprofit homes are usually governed through a board of directors or advisory group and do not pay out any profits to owners or investors. The majority of homes (over 80%) are proprietary and operated as a business that is expected to provide a profit to the owners. Some are independent, while others operate as part of a chain. Both types of nursing homes must be licensed by the state and conform to standards set by state and local laws. In order to receive Medicare or Medicaid payments, the homes must also meet federal standards. The type of ownership makes a difference, not necessarily in standards of care, but in who makes major decisions regarding the policies, staff, and programs of the facility.

Although there is no direct relationship between size and quality of care, size is an important nursing home characteristic to consider in relation to the older person's preferences and the availability of needed services. Although smaller facilities may be more personal and homelike and better able to respond to individual needs, larger facilities often have more resources and amenities as well as a wider range of specialized services. Regardless of size, important considerations are the ratio of staff (registered nurses [RNs] and certified nurse assistants [CNAs]) to residents, whether there is a physician on staff and an in-house pharmacy, and whether the particular services needed will be available.

Location is one of the most important selection factors. Accessibility of the home to family members and friends, especially those who are most committed to the older person and likely to have the most time for visiting, can mean the difference between frequent and infrequent visitors. Geographical uprooting should always be a last resort, but may be necessary to achieve this kind of accessibility for the family member(s) who will maintain the closest ties with the older person. If the person will be entering a nursing home in the same area and wishes to continue to be cared for by the same primary care provider, that physician should be contacted to determine which nursing homes he or she is willing to visit. Many physicians prefer to have patients in only one or a few nursing homes for their convenience and efficient use of their time.

These considerations should help the older person and/or family members to narrow down the choices and select several homes for a preplacement observation visit to ascertain how well each home matches the individual's preferences and lifestyle. They are consumers shopping for a product—nursing home care—and they have a right to know what they will be purchasing. The person responsible for admissions in each home (usually the administrator, director of nursing services, or social worker) should be contacted to arrange for a tour of the facility. Any home that is not willing to cooperate with a preplacement visit should be crossed off the list.

It is particularly important to inquire about nurse staffing. Questions about staffing should focus on the credentials of the staff, staff stability, and the ratio of professional to nonprofessional staff. The director of nursing should have special preparation in care of the elderly and several years' experience in nursing homes. Similarly, the registered professional staff should be experienced in gerontological nursing. Certification in gerontological nursing by the American Nurses Association is one indication of adherence to high professional standards; nurse aide certification is another indicator of high standards.

Staff stability can be determined by inquiring how long the present and prior director of nursing have been in the home, turnover of other professional staff, and the percentage of staff who are part-time (agency workers) rather than employees of the home. High turnover may indicate administrative instability and/or discontent with care on the part of staff. Older people and their families should know to inquire about the ratio of professional (RN) nurse staff to nursing aides or assistants. Studies suggest that the higher the professional staff mix the better the care (Specter & Takada, 1991). Lastly, quality of care has been shown to be high in homes which employ nurses with advanced preparation as geriatric nurse practitioners and clinicians (Mezey, 1991; Garrard, Kane, Ratner, & Buchanon, 1991).

It is recommended that the older person and/or family member(s) make a list of areas they would like to see, including the kitchen, dining areas, patient rooms, bathroom facilities, activity rooms, and lounges. Although cleanliness and modernity may make a good first impression, a place that seems homey and comfortable to the older person may have greater livability in the long run. Table 13.4 includes questions regarding comfort inside the facility, appearance and activities of the residents, staff and resident interactions, appearance of resident's rooms, and outside environment. They can be used to guide the observations of the older person and/or family member(s) as they make their tour and help them to judge the quality of each nursing home as a place to live.

In addition to evaluating the livability of the nursing home environment, the older person and/or family member(s) should be guided to evaluate the programs offered. Table 13.5 includes questions that can direct the thinking of the visitors during the tour about things that will be important to the prospective resident concerning food service, activities, policies about the use of physical and chemical restraints, use of advance directives (living wills and health care proxys), community outreach, resident participation, and family participation. Because nursing homes can differ significantly, careful consideration must be given to the match between the older person's needs and preferences and each of these service areas in the facilities being considered.

During the visit, in addition to ascertaining that the building and grounds are well-maintained, environmental design features that compensate for age changes and that promote functional independence and safety can be noted. These features can include:

1. use of bright, warm colors with sharp contrasts (for example, on doors and door frames, baseboards, stair edges, etc.) to enhance visual discrimination
2. fabric or horizontal louvered shades that block bright sunshine but admit natural light, as well as adequate shielding for bright lights to reduce glare and concentrated light on work areas, doorways, and floors to reduce shadows
3. nonreflective, nonslip flooring (note: geriatric patients have been found to prefer carpeting which makes the environment quieter,

**TABLE 13.4 Questions about the Livability of a Nursing Home**

Comfort of the facility:

Is the temperature reasonable? Is the air free of strong odors, such as stale food, urine, or cleaning products? Is the noise level pleasant? A good home will usually have a rather constant hum of activity, with occasional outbursts from laughter or conversation.

Appearance of the residents:

Try to see past the fact that many of the residents are in a state of declining mental or physical health and require walkers, canes, and wheelchairs. Instead, look at whether they are generally neat and comfortably dressed. Do they have clean hair, clean hands, and trimmed fingernails?

Activity of the residents:

Are residents in their rooms or are they active in various parts of the home? Are there indications of activity and efforts to relate to the residents—such as large-print calendars and posters on the walls, current magazines and newspapers, displays of crafts, etc. Is there a house pet? Do the residents have a newsletter?

Interactions between staff and residents:

Are staff members generally available to the residents? Do they seem to be naturally friendly and courteous both to you as a visitor and to the residents? Are staff members neat in their appearance? Do staff members speak the language of your relative?

Appearance of patient rooms:

Are the rooms kept clean? Is there adequate space for your relative to feel comfortable? Are most of the rooms for one, two, or three persons? Do the rooms seem homey?

Impression of the outside environment:

Are there places to walk or sit outside? Is there activity that can be observed from the windows? Are the grounds kept up nicely? Are there any resources nearby, such as a library or senior center that your relative might enjoy? Is the neighborhood safe?

From: *Choosing a nursing home: A guidebook for families*, by the Pacific Northwest Long-Term Care Council, 1985. Seattle: University of Washington. Reprinted with permission.

reduces glare, increases sturdiness of footing, and reduces fear of falling)

4. presence of handrails along corridor walls, ramps instead of stairs, and levers on doors that are easier to manipulate than round knobs
5. furniture that is user friendly (for example, chairs with wide arm rests, short seats, and high backs to allow ease of standing and pedestal tables that lessen the risk of tripping and facilitate movements of walkers and wheelchairs), covered with bright, washable, interestingly textured fabrics, and arranged in modular

**TABLE 13.5 Questions for Evaluating Programs Offered by Nursing Home**

Food service

What is the menu for the current week and how often is it repeated? How are food preferences of the residents recognized/incorporated into the menu? Are refreshments available to residents and guests in between meals? Is the Dining room atmosphere pleasant and friendly? Do residents have a choice of where and with whom they sit? Can residents have guests for dinner? What are the policies regarding meal service to the rooms, late or early meals, availability of snacks, and food storage in the rooms?

Activities

What therapy programs are offered? What are the credentials of the therapists? How often is each type of therapy available? What kind of social/recreational programs are offered and how often? What opportunities are there for participation in religious services? (Ask to see current month's activity schedule.)

Community outreach

To what extent are residents able to maintain previous connections with the community? Does the home provide outings to senior centers, shopping excursions, volunteer work sites? Are residents taken for supervised walks? Do volunteers from community organizations come into the home to encourage resident participation in various activities? Could a resident maintain active membership in a community group by attending meetings outside and/or having the group meet at the nursing home occasionally?

Resident participation

How are residents involved in decision-making about things that affect their lifestyle and well-being? Is there an active resident council, suggestion box, or resident participation on the board? What mechanisms are available to residents to make a complaint or express a concern? Is there an impartial method for settling differences? Is the "Resident Bill of Rights" explained and made available to all residents?

Family participation

Does the home invite families to social events? Encourage families to participate in resident programs? Plan special outings for residents and their families? Are family members encouraged to participate in development of the care plan? Is the family contacted routinely when unusual progress is made or problems arise? Are there mechanisms such as a family council, family conferences, newsletter, or family support group that indicate a policy of promoting family involvement?

*Note*: Adapted from *Choosing a nursing home: A guidebook for families*, by the Pacific Northwest Long-Term Care Council, 1985. Seattle: University of Washington.

patterns that facilitate social interaction rather than a "park bench" type of line-up

6. adaptation of the environment to wheelchairs (if applicable), for example, lowered pictures, light switches, shelves, and drawers as well as beds, chairs, desks, tables, sinks and toilets at wheelchair height (Andreasen, 1985).

In addition, the prospective nursing home resident and/or family member(s) should also request to see the facility license and a copy of the admission agreement and to ask specific questions about the following:

1. admission standards (which define the type of resident population)
2. discharge policies
3. monetary arrangements
4. room assignments and changes (including whether residents have any choice about room location or roommates)
5. policies regarding holding rooms if residents are hospitalized or take a vacation
6. policies concerning the amount and type of personal possessions that can be brought in
7. care of valuables and precautions against theft
8. policies/procedures to protect the privacy of residents
9. visiting hours and administrative flexibility in unusual circumstances
10. policies/schedule regarding bedtime, mealtime, and frequency of bathing (compared to prospective resident's lifestyle)
11. procedures for dealing with emergencies and life-threatening illness.

Policies regarding pets may also be of interest to the potential nursing home resident.

According to Kastenbaum (1981), too much habituation and too little control tend to undermine adaptation and fulfillment in old age and can lead to individuals becoming doubly (both chronologically and psychologically) old. In nursing homes with overly ritualized and constant environments, even cognitively intact residents are at risk for "hyperhabituation," a syndrome characterized by: a routinized sense of time and a repetitive, fixed sequence of activities that render the individual unable to adapt flexibly to new situations; a "nothing new here" outlook that induces mental stagnation; disinterest in meeting new people and in getting involved with others; constriction of the range of one's physical and social environment (for example, staying in one's room, seldom participating in group activities or trips); and being a passive participant in activities (a watcher rather than a doer).

It is important to judge whether there is evidence in the nursing home(s) under consideration of planned variety or encouragement of spontaneous changes in environmental stimuli and activities that will reduce the risk of hyperhabitulation and whether efforts are made to reverse this kind of response in residents who manifest these behaviors (Norris-Baker & Scheidt, 1989).

Before the final decision is made, it is advisable for the older person and/or family member(s) to further check out the nursing home that is their first choice to see if their positive impressions are reinforced by the experience/opinions of others. Another informal unannounced visit to the home may be helpful, during which resident/ staff interaction can be more closely observed and residents and their families asked about what living in the home is really like. The additional information gathered from these observations will help the older person and/or family members to judge whether the setting is one which will decrease or reinforce disability, and foster or diminish the dignity, self-reliance, control, and decision-making abilities that are essential for a fulfilling life at any age.

In summary, although nursing homes are regulated by the same federal and state authorities, their general atmosphere, programs, and policies vary. Once the choice of homes has been narrowed down, the final decision should be based on how well the home matches the older person's physical and psychosocial needs. Major consideration should be given to the individual's need for: closeness to family, friends, and primary care providers; specific treatments and/or physical, mental, and social activity; and a living arrangement that accommodates to his or her personal habits, preferences, and lifestyle.

## NURSING IMPLICATIONS

Knowledge of common normal age changes and health deviations can be very helpful to the nurse in assessing the interaction of older people with their environment. In particular many features of the home and community have a significant impact on the health and well-being of the noninstitutionalized elderly. This chapter has attempted to describe aspects of the community and home environment that can be particularly helpful or detrimental to an older person's efforts to maintain independence.

The practitioner can utilize the data gathered during a home visit to assess the adequacy of the client's environment in meeting his or her needs. In collaboration with the older person, the practitioner can help the client gain access to needed community resources and services, or enhance comfort, security, and safety within the home and neighborhood. For example, some recommendations that may be useful to promote the safety of an older person with dementia would include: removing the bathroom door lock; keeping the fireplace (if any) screened, and locking up matches, sharp objects and chemicals (for example, cleaning products); removing the knobs from the stove or shutting off its electrical circuit breaker; disconnecting the garbage disposal and installing drain traps in the sinks; keeping the entrances to the basement, attic, utility room, and garage locked; and arranging for live-in caregiver(s) to have their own private space in the home which can be locked and provide them a place of respite.

The nurse's assessment may lead to the judgment that the older person cannot be maintained adequately in the present environment. Helping this older person and his or her family to identify and accept more appropriate housing or services, and making referrals to initiate this change, are an important part of the nursing process. There should then be follow-up to ensure continuity of care and to facilitate adjustment to the new environment. Even when the nurse is unable to visit the home and neighborhood directly, it is important to have an awareness of the value of this kind of assessment in providing a more complete picture of the client's health status. This awareness will motivate the practitioner to obtain as much data as possible indirectly, from the client or family, as part of the health history.

## ACKNOWLEDGMENT

This chapter was reviewed by Jan Grossnickle, RN, BSN, of Sharp Home Health Care and Sharp Senior Healthcare's Geriatric Evaluation and Management (GEM) Program, San Diego, CA. Her wise insights and practical suggestions gained from extensive experience with home and community assessment of frail elderly clients have enriched the revision and expansion of this chapter.

## REFERENCES

Andreasen, M. A. K. (1985). Make a safe environment by design. *Journal of Gerontological Nursing, 11*(6), 18–22.

Bernardin-Haldeman, V. (1988). Ecology and aging: A critical review. *Canadian Journal on Aging, 7*(4), 458–471.

Evans, G. W., Brennan, P. L., Skorpanich, M. A., & Held, D. (1984). Cognitive mapping and elderly adults: Verbal and location memory for urban landmarks. *Journal of Gerontology, 39*(4), 452–457.

Garrard, J., Kane, R., Ratner, E., & Buchanon, J. (1991). The impact of nurse practitioners on the care of nursing home residents. In Katz, P., Kane, R., & Mezey, M. *Advances in long-term care.* Volume 1, (pp. 169–183). New York: Springer Publishing Co.

Golant, S. M. (1986). Understanding the diverse housing environments of the elderly. *Environments, 18*(3), 35–51.

Harootyan, R. (1988). Improving environmental design technologies for the elderly. *American Behavioral Scientist, 31*(5), 607–613.

Kahana, E. (1982). A congruence model of person-environment interaction. In Lawton, M. P., Windley, P. G., & Byerts, T. O. (Eds.), *Aging and the environment: Theoretical approaches* (pp. 97–121). New York: Springer Publishing Co.

Kastenbaum, R. (1981). Habituation as a model of human aging. *International Journal of Aging and Human Development, 12*(3), 159–170.

Kay, A. D., & Tideiksaar, L. (1990). Falls and gait disorders. In Abrams, W. B., & Berkow, R. (Eds.), *The Merck manual of geriatrics* (p. 52). Rahway, NJ: Merck, Sharp & Dohme.

Kemper, P., & Murtaugh, C. M. (1991). Lifetime use of nursing home care. *New England Journal of Medicine, 324*(112), 595–600.

Lawton, M. P. (1987a). Environment and the need satisfaction of the aging. In Carstensen, L. L., & Edelstein, B. A. (Eds.), *Handbook of clinical gerontology* (pp. 33–40). New York: Pergamon Press.

Lawton, M. P. (1987b). Aging and proactivity in the residential environment. Paper presented at the annual meeting of the American Psychological Association, Division of Community Psychology, New York City, September 1, 1987.

Lawton, M. P. (1980). Environmental change: The older person as initiator and responder. In Datan, N., & Lohmann, N. (Eds.), *Transitions of aging.* New York: Academic Press.

Lawton, M. P., & Nahemow, L. (1973). Ecology and the aging process. In Eisdorfer, C., & Lawton, M. P. (Eds.), *Psychology of adult development and aging* (pp. 619–674). Washington, DC: American Psychological Association.

Lawton, M. P., & Simon, B. (1968). The ecology of social relationships in housing for the elderly. *Gerontologist, 8,* 108–115.

Mezey, M. (1991). Nursing homes: Residents' needs; nursing's response. In Aiken, L., & Fagin, C. (Eds.), *Charting nursing's future: Agenda for the 1990s* (pp. 198–216). Philadelphia: J.B. Lippincott.

Norris-Baker, C., & Scheidt, R. J. (1989). Habituation theory and environment-aging research: Ennui to joie de vivre? *International Journal of Aging and Human Development, 29*(4), 241–257.

Pacific Northwest Long-Term Care Council. (1985). *Choosing a nursing home.* Seattle: University of Washington.

Rowles, G. D. (1984). The surveillance zone as meaningful space for the aged. *The Gerontologist, 21*(3), 304–311.

Saperstein, A., Lawton, M. P., Moleski, W. H., & Sharp, A. (1984). *A housing quality component for in-home services.* Philadelphia: Philadelphia Operation for the Aging.

Slack, P. (1986, Sept. 17). Home hunting. *Nursing Times,* 29–30.

Spector, W. D., & Takada, H. A. (1991). Characteristics of nursing homes that affect resident outcomes. *Journal of Aging and Health, 3*(4), 427–454.

Staab, A. S., & Lyles, M. A. (1990). *Manual of geriatric nursing* (p. 5). Glenview, IL: Scott, Foresman & Co.

Werner, C. M., Altman, I., & Oxley, D. (1985). Temporal aspects of home: A transactional analysis. In Altman, I. & Werner, C. M. (Eds.), *Home environments.* New York: Plenum.

Wister, A. V. (1989). Environmental adaptation by persons in their later life. *Research on Aging, 11*(3), 267–291.

## SUGGESTED READINGS

Altman, I., Lawton, M. P., & Wohlwill, J. F. (Eds.). (1984). *Elderly people and the environment.* New York: Plenum.

Altman, I., & Werner, C. M. (1985). Home environments. New York: Plenum.

Beland, F. (1987). Living preferences among elderly people. *The Gerontologist, 27*(6), 797–803.

Borgata, E. F., & Montgomery, R. J. V. (Eds.). (1987). *Critical issues in aging policy.* Newbury Park, CA: Sage.

Buttimer, A., & Seamon, D. (Eds.). (1984). *The human experience of space and place.* London: Croom Helm.

Carstensen, L. L., & Edelstein, B. A. (Eds.). (1987). *Handbook of clinical gerontology.* New York: Pergamon Press.

Chellis, R. D. et al. (Eds.). (1982). *Congregate housing for older people: A solution for the 1980s.* Lexington, MA: Lexington Press.

Datan, N., & Lohmann, N. (Eds.). (1980). *Transitions of aging.* New York: Academic Press.

Fisher, J. D., Bell, P., & Baum, W. (Eds.). (1984). *Environmental psychology* (2nd ed.). NY: Holt, Rhinehart & Winston.

Hiatt, L. G. (1986). The environment's role in the total well-being of the older person. In Magan, G. G., & Haught, E. L. (Eds.), *Well being and the elderly* (pp. 23–37). Washington, DC: American Association of Homes for the Aging.

Holahan, C. J. (1982). *Environmental psychology.* New York: Random House.

Howell, S. C. (1980). *Designing for aging: Patterns of use.* Cambridge, MA: MIT Press.

Jarvik, L., & Small, G. (1988). *Parentcare: A commonsense guide for adult children* (2nd ed.). New York: Crown Publishers.

Kane, R. L., Ouslander, J. G., & Abrass, I. B. (1989). *Essentials of clinical geriatrics* (2nd ed.). New York: McGraw-Hill.

Kaufman, S. (1986). *The ageless self: Sources of meaning in late life.* Madison, WI: University of Wisconsin Press.

Kinney, S. M., Stephens, M. A. P., & Brockmann, A. M. (1987). Personal and environmental correlates of territoriality and use of space: An illustration in congregate housing for older adults. *Environment and Behavior, 19*(6), 722–737.

Lawton, M. P. (1980). *Environment and aging.* Monterey, CA: Brooks/Cole Publishing Co.

Lawton, M. P. (1983). Environment and other determinants of well-being in older people. *Gerontologist, 23,* 349–357.

Lawton, M. P., Windley, P. G., & Byerts, T. O. (Eds.). (1982). *Aging and the environment: Theoretical approaches.* New York: Springer Publishing Co.

Lesnoff-Caravaglia, G. (1987). *Handbook of applied gerontology.* New York: Human Sciences Press, Inc.

O'Bryant, S. L. (1983). The subjective value of "home" to older homeowners. *Journal of Housing for the Elderly, 1,* 29–43.

Rowles, G. D. (1981). Geographical perspectives on human development. *Human Development, 24,* 67–76.

Rowles, G. D., & Ohta, R. J. (Eds.). (1983). *Aging and milieu.* New York: Academic Press.

Rubenstein, R. L. (1987). The significance of personal objects to older people. *Journal of Aging Studies, 1,* 226–238.

Rubenstein, R. L. (1989). The home environments of older people: A description of the psycho-social processes linking person to place. *Journal of Gerontology, 44*(2), S45–S53.

Silverstone, B., & Hyman, H. K. (1982). *You and your aging parent: A modern family's guide to emotional, physical, and financial problems.* New York: Pantheon Books.

Stephens, M. A. P., Kinney, J. M., & McNeer, A. E. (1986). Accommodative housing: Social integration among well and frail residents. *Gerontologist, 26,* 176–180.

Torres-Stanovik, R. (Ed.). (1990). *Caregiver's handbook.* San Diego, CA: San Diego County Mental Health Services.

U.S. Congress, Office of Technology Assessment. (1985). *Technology and aging in America.* (OTA-BA-264). Washington, DC: U.S. Government Printing Office.

# **14**

# Changes in Laboratory Values and Their Implications

Despite significant decreases in organ system function in healthy older persons (for example, a 40% decrease in lung vital capacity and a 30% decrease in cardiac output), there may be only a slight alteration in most laboratory test results during a resting state. More markedly abnormal findings may result, however, when dynamic tests of organ functional reserve are administered to healthy elderly individuals (Rock, 1984, p. 57), for example while a fasting plasma glucose level may be normal or only slightly elevated, plasma glucose levels 1 and 2 hours after concentrated glucose ingestion may be significantly elevated.

Careful interpretation of appropriate laboratory values is a particularly important aspect of assessment of the health state of older persons because the ill elderly frequently present with vague or atypical clinical signs and symptoms. When reviewing laboratory test results seen in the elderly, it is necessary to consider whether any reported values that are outside the normal ranges reflect illness, iatrogenic causes (for example, medications), or normal age changes. Most reference intervals published in standard textbooks and laboratory handbooks are derived from studies of subjects aged 20 to 40. Since the 1970s, numerous studies of random samples of "healthy" individuals have been done to begin to establish age-related normal laboratory values. However, since a majority of the elderly have one or more disease entities and are taking one or more medications, it is difficult to define healthy elderly populations for the purpose of developing normal laboratory values for this age group (Dever & Rothkopf, 1990, p. 101).

According to Kane, Oslander, and Abrass (1989), misinterpretation of an abnormal laboratory value as an age change can lead to underdiagnosis and undertreatment of some conditions (for example, anemia), while failure to appreciate age-related changes in normal laboratory values can lead to overdiagnosis and overtreatment of other conditions (for example, hyperglycemia). Therefore, laboratory value changes due to aging must be distinguished from pathologic changes related to disease or alterations due to the effects of medications and/or other treatment modalities. While a slightly abnormal laboratory value should not be interpreted as definite evidence of disease, a normal value does not necessarily rule out a disease (Burrage, Dixon, & Sehy, 1991).

This chapter presents an overview of laboratory values that significantly change with aging. Whenever possible, the reason(s) for the observed laboratory value changes is discussed; however, some observed changes are not yet completely understood. Table 14.1 summarizes normal age-related changes in standard reference range values for frequently used tests, and common causes of deviations from normal laboratory values. Normal standard reference range values vary with different clinical laboratories. Therefore the practitioner should refer to the normal range parameters of the laboratory used in his or her agency/institution when interpreting test results. It should be noted that sex differences in the normal ranges for many tests change with aging; some differences develop or persist into old age, while others become clinically insignificant.

## HEMATOLOGY

Aging itself has less effect on hematopoiesis than socioeconomic factors and physical limitations; for example, poverty, inadequate nutrition, and impaired mobility may be associated with a reduction in the number of circulating red blood cells, granulocytes, and lymphocytes (Andres, Bierman, & Hazzard, 1985).

### Red Blood Cell Indices

There is little evidence of age-related differences in red blood cells (RBCs). Changes in red cell enzymes that cause a slight increase in mean cell diameter have been documented, but the blood volume remains constant (Dever & Rothkopf, 1990, p. 104). By age 70 there is a 40% decline in bone

**TABLE 14.1. Laboratory Values in the Elderly and Their Implications**

| | Standard reference values* alterations in SRVs | | Clinical implications of deviations+ | |
|---|---|---|---|---|
| Tests | (SRVs) for adults | With normal aging | Increased levels | Decreased levels |
| Hematology Hemoglobin | M: 13.5–18 g/dL<br>F: 12–16 g/dL | Slight ↓ (M>F); values in both sexes more nearly the same | High altitude<br>Dehydration<br>Polycythemia<br>Advanced COPD<br>CHF<br>Severe burns | Fluid overload<br>Anemias<br>Cancers<br>Chronic renal failures<br>Fluid overload |
| Hematocrit | M: 40–54%<br>F: 36–46% | Slight ↓ in males | Dehydration<br>Polycythemia<br>Diabetic acidosis<br>Trauma, surgery, burns<br>Late stage emphysema | Hemorrhage<br>Anemias<br>Leukemias<br>Lymphomas<br>Liver & kidney diseases<br>Malnutrition<br>Collagen diseases |
| RBCs | M:4.6–6.0<br>F: 4.0–5.0 | Unchanged | Dehydration<br>Polycythemia<br>High altitude<br>Advanced COPD | Fluid overload<br>Hemorrhage<br>Anemias<br>Leukemias<br>Chronic infections<br>Chronic renal failure |
| MCV | 80–98 | Slight ↑ | Macrocytic anemias<br>Chronic liver disease<br>Anticonvulsants &<br>anti-metabolite drugs | Microcytic anemias<br>Malignancy<br>Rheumatoid arthritis<br>Hemoglobinopathies<br>Lead poisoning<br>Radiation |

*(continued)*

**TABLE 14.1.** (*continued*)

| Tests | Standard reference values* (SRVs) for adults | With normal aging | Clinical implications of deviations+ | |
|---|---|---|---|---|
| | | | Increased levels | Decreased levels |
| MCH | 27–31 | Unchanged | Macrocytic anemias | Microcytic, hypochromic anemia (Fe deficiency) |
| MCHC | 32–36% | Unchanged | | Hypochromic anemias (Fe deficiency & thalassemia) |
| Erythrocyte Sedimentation Rate (ESR) | Westergren Method: M: 0–10 mm/h F: 0–20 mm/h | Slight ↑ in both sexes M: 0–20 mm/h F: 0–30 mm/h | Acute MI SLE + RA Malignancy Bacterial infections Gout Surgery, burns | Polycythemia CHF Sickle cell anemia Degenerative arthritis Factor V deficiency |
| Total WBC | 4,500–10,000/cu mm | # Unchanged, but ↓ function | Acute infections Tissue necrosis (acute MI) Collagen diseases Parasitic diseases Stress | Hematopoietic diseases Viral infections Alcoholism SLE, RA |
| WBC Differential -Neutrophils | Total 50–70% Segs 50–65% Bands 0–5% | # Unchanged, but may be less effective bone marrow response to acute infection | Acute infections Inflammatory diseases Tissue damage Hodgkin's disease | Viral diseases Leukemias BM depression |
| -Lymphocytes | 25–35% | # Unchanged but ↓ in both B & T cell function and ↑ in autoantibody production | Acute viral infections Chronic bact. infection Lymphocytic leukemia Hodgkins, mult. myeloma | Cancer Leukemia BM depression Multiple sclerosis Renal disease |

210

| | | | | |
|---|---|---|---|---|
| | | | Adrenocortical hypofunction | SLE, Adrenocortical hyperfunction |
| -Monocytes | 4–6% | Slight ↑ in both sexes | Viral & parasitic diseases, Cancer, Monocytic leukemia, Collagen diseases | Lymphocytic leukemia, Aplastic anemia |
| -Eosinophils | 1–3% | Unchanged | Allergies, Parasitic diseases, Cancer, Thrombophlebitis | Stress (burns, shock), Adrenocortical hyperfunction |
| -Basophils | 0.4–1.0% | Unchanged | Healing stage of infection/inflammation, Leukemia | Stress, Hypersensitivity reaction |
| Blood Gases | | | | |
| Arterial pH | 7.35–7.45 | Unchanged | Respiratory or metabolic alkalosis, Na bicarbonate, Na or K oxalate | Respiratory or metabolic acidosis, Narcotics, barbiturates, acetazolamide or ammonium chloride |
| Pa $O_2$ | 75–100 mg Hg. | Gradual ↓ | | Respiratory or cardiac disease |
| Pa $CO_2$ | 35–45 mm Hg. | Unchanged or slight ↑ with advancing age | Respiratory acidosis | Respiratory alkalosis |

(continued)

**TABLE 14.1.** (*continued*)

| | Standard reference values* alterations in SRVs | | Clinical implications of deviations+ | |
|---|---|---|---|---|
| Tests | (SRVs) for adults | With normal aging | Increased levels | Decreased levels |
| **Serum Chemistries** | | | | |
| Iron | 50–150 µg/dL (2–3 x serum Fe level) | ↓ to 50–75% young adult value by 7th decade | Pernicious hemolytic & folic acid deficiency anemias Hemochromatosis Liver damage Thalassemia Lead toxicity | Fe deficiency anemia Chronic blood loss GI malignancies Peptic ulcer Rheumatoid arthritis Chronic renal failure |
| Total Iron Binding Capacity (TIBC) | 250–450 µg/dL 2–3 x serum Fe level) | TIBC ↓ while % transferrin saturation unchanged at 25–30% | Fe deficiency anemia Acute/chronic blood loss Polycythemia | Hemolytic, pernicious, sickle cell anemias Hemochromatosis Renal failure Liver disease Rheumatoid arthritis GI malignancies |
| Ferritin | 12–300 µg/dL | Unchanged (more sensitive indicator of Fe deficiency than Serum Fe) | Hemochromatosis | Fe deficiency anemia |
| $B_{12}$ | 200–900 pg/dL | ↓ to 60–80% young adult value by 7th decade | Acute hepatitis Myelocytic leukemia Polycythemia | Inadequate intake Pernicious anemia Malabsorption syndrome Sprue Pancreatic insufficiency Gastrectomy Liver disease Crohn's disease |

| Test | Normal Values | Changes with Age | Increased | Decreased |
|---|---|---|---|---|
| Folic Acid (folate) | 3–16 ng/mL (bioassay)<br>>2.5 ng/mL (radioimmunoassay)<br>>200–700 mg/mL (RBC) | Unchanged | Pernicious anemia | Malnutrition<br>Folic acid or B$_6$ deficiency anemia<br>Liver disease<br>ETOH, sulfa drugs, anticonvulsants<br>Malabsorption syndromes |
| **Glucose**<br>Fasting plasma glucose (FPG) | 70–110 mg/dL | 70–120 mg/dL or ↑ 2 mg/dL/decade after age 35 | Uncontrolled diabetes mellitus<br>Hyperadrenalism<br>Stress, infections, burns<br>Acute pancreatitis<br>Extensive surgery<br>Thiazides | Malnutrition<br>Alcoholism<br>Strenuous exercise<br>Hypoglycemic reaction (insulin shock)<br>Cancer of stomach, liver or lung<br>Hypoadrenalism<br>Cirrhosis of liver |
| Post prandial plasma glucose (PPPG) | <140 mg/dL<br>2 hr after meal | <160 mg/dL/2 hr | | |
| Oral glucose tolerance test (OGTT) | <u>Plasma values:</u><br>Fasting 70–110 mg/dL<br>0.5 hr < 160 mg/dL<br>1 hr < 170 mg/dL<br>2 hrs < 125 mg/dL<br>3 hr fasting level | Fasting plasma glucose ↑ more quickly in the first 2 hours, then ↓ to baseline more slowly<br>1 hr plasma glucose ↓ 4–14 md/dL/decade after age 35 | ↓ glucose tolerance<br>Diabetes mellitus–latent or overt<br>Insulin resistance<br>Hyperadrenalism<br>Stress, infections, extensive surgery or injury<br>Cancer of pancreas<br>Intense stress<br>Sedentary lifestyle with high fat diet | Hyperinsulinism<br>Hypoadrenalism<br>Malabsorption<br>Protein malnutrition |

*(continued)*

213

**TABLE 14.1.** (*continued*)

| Tests | Standard reference values* alterations in SRVs | | Clinical implications of deviations+ | |
| | (SRVs) for adults | With normal aging | Increased levels | Decreased levels |
|---|---|---|---|---|
| Cholesterol | < 200/mg/dL | ↑ in males to age 50, then ↓ in females to age 50, then ↑ to 70 and ↓ after 70 | Hyperlipoproteinemia<br>Atherosclerosis<br>Uncontrolled diabetes mellitus<br>Hypothroidism<br>Cirrhosis of liver<br>Nephrotic syndrome | Hyperthyroidism<br>Starvation<br>Malabsorption |
| HDL fraction | > 45 mg/dL = low risk | Females higher than males until 7th decade | ↓ CV risk | ↑ CV risk |
| Total Serum Proteins | 6.0–8.0 g/dL | Unchanged | Dehydration<br>Severe vomiting &/or diarrhea | Severe malnutrition<br>Cirrhosis, liver failure<br>Severe burns<br>Renal disease<br>Certain malignancies<br>Ulcerative colitis<br>Malabsorption or protein losing GI diseases |
| Albumin | 3.5–5 g/dL<br>52–68% of total protein | Slight ↓ (< 0.5 mg/dL) Before 65, levels ↑ in males; after 65, values equalize and ↓ | | |
| Uric Acid | M: 3.5–8 mg/dL<br>F: 2.8–6.8 mg/dL | Male values remain higher than females throughout life, but female values ↑ in 4th or 5th decade | Gout<br>Alcoholism<br>Metastatic cancer<br>Leukemias, multiple myeloma, lymphoma<br>Hyperlipoproteinomia<br>Glomerulonephritis<br>Renal failure<br>CHF<br>Hemolytic anemia<br>Polycythemia | Folic acid, anemia<br>Wilson's disease<br>Renal tubular acidosis<br>Burns |

214

| | Normal Value | Age-Related Changes | | |
|---|---|---|---|---|
| Blood Urea Nitrogen | 5–25 mg/dL | Slight ↑ in both sexes with lower average values in females | Dehydration<br>High protein intake<br>Acute MI<br>Prerenal failure<br>Renal disease<br>GI bleeding<br>Sepsis<br>Diabetes mellitus<br>Excessive ingestion of licorice | Overhydration<br>Low protein diet<br>Sever liver damage |
| Creatinine | 0.5–1.5 mg/dL<br>(Females may have slightly lower values due to less muscle mass) | May ↑ slightly, but varies little with age despite ↓ renal function due to ↓ muscle mass and ↓ production in the muscles | Diet high in meat/fish (usually minimal effect)<br>Renal failure<br>Prolonged shock<br>Acute MI<br>Cancers<br>SLE | |
| Creatinine Clearance (urine) | 85–135 ml/min<br>(Females may have slightly lower values) | Progressive ↓ in both sexes | Diabetic nephropathy<br>Renovascular hyper-tension<br>Hypothyroidism<br>Exercise | Renal impairment<br>Hyperthyroidism<br>Muscular dystrophy<br>Amyotrophic lateral sclerosis |
| Serum Electrolytes:<br>Potassium | 3.5–5.0 mEq/L | Slight age-related ↑ after 6th decade | Renal failure<br>Hyperadrenalism<br>Metabolic acidosis | Vomiting/diarrhea<br>Laxative abuse<br>Dehydration<br>Starvation<br>Stress<br>Traumatic injury & surgery<br>Metabolic alkalosis<br>Burns<br>Hyperaldosteronism |

*(continued)*

215

# TABLE 14.1. (continued)

| Tests | Standard reference values* (SRVs) for adults | With normal aging | Clinical implications of deviations+ | |
|---|---|---|---|---|
| | | | Increased levels | Decreased levels |
| Other serum electrolytes | | Unchanged | | |
| Serum Enzymes– Alkaline Phosphatase (ALP) | 20–90 IU/L @ 30°C (SI units) | Slight gradual ↑ in both sexes with greater ↑ in females | Obstructive liver disease<br>Cancer of bone, breast, prostate<br>Leukemia, mult. myeloma<br>Pagets disease<br>Healing fractures | Hypothyroidism<br>Malnutrition<br>Vitamin C deficiency<br>Hypophosphatasia<br>Pernicious anemia |
| Creatine Phosphokinase (CPK) | M: 5–35 μg/mL<br>F: 5–25 μg/mL | May not be elevated in acute MI (so important to measure CPK-MB isoenzyme) | Acute MI<br>Skeletal muscle disease<br>CVA | |
| CPK Isoenzymes | CPK-MM 94–100% (muscle) | Muscular dystrophy | Delirium tremens<br>Crush injury/trauma<br>Surgery<br>Vigorous exercise<br>Hypokalemia | |
| | CPK-MB 0–6% (heart) | | Acute MI<br>Cardiac ischemia<br>Hypokalemia<br>Cardiac-surgery | |

216

| Test | Normal Value | Age-Related Change | Increased In | Decreased In |
|---|---|---|---|---|
| | CPK-BB 0% (brain) | | CVA<br>Brain cancer<br>Brain injury<br>Pulmonary infarction | |
| Gamma Glutamyl Transpeptidase (GGT) | 0–45 IU/L (overall avg)<br>M: 10–80 IU/L<br>F: –5–25 IU/L | Slight ↑ in females | Liver disease<br>Alcoholism<br>Many cancers<br>Renal disease<br>Acute MI (4th day)<br>CHF<br>Acute pancreatitis | |

**Hormone Levels**

Thyroid Indices:

| Test | Normal Value | Age-Related Change | Increased In | Decreased In |
|---|---|---|---|---|
| T₄ | T₄ by column 4.5–11.5 µg/dL T₄RIA 5–12 µg/dL Free T₄ 1.0–2.3 mg/dL | Slight ↓ (up to 25%) | Hyperthyroidism<br>Acute thyroiditis<br>Viral hepatitis<br>Myesthenia gravis | Hypothyroidism<br>Protein malnutrition<br>Ant. pituitary hypofunction<br>Strenuous exercise<br>Renal failure |
| T₃ | T₃RIA 80–200 mg/dL | ↓ in males after age 60<br>↓ in females after age 70 or 80 | Hyperthyroidism<br>T₃ thyrotoxicosis<br>Hashimoto's thyroiditis<br>Toxic thyroid adenoma | Severe illness or trauma<br>Malnutrition |
| TSH | 2–5.4 µIU/mL | ↑ in both sexes after age 60 | Primary hypothyroidism<br>Hashimotos thyroiditis<br>Antithyroid drug therapy | Hyperthyroidism<br>Hypothyroidism due to pituitary insufficiency |
| Thyroid Releasing Hormone (TRH) Stimulation Test | 15–30 min after TRH administration TSH levels should rise 2.5 to 4x baseline & return to baseline in 2–4 hr. | ↓ in expected TSH surge in healthy older men | Primary hypothroidism | Primary hypopituitarism<br>Autonomous thyroid hyperactivity |

*(continued)*

**TABLE 14.1.** (*continued*)

| Tests | Standard reference values* alterations in SRVs (SRVs) for adults | With normal aging | Clinical implications of deviations+ Increased levels | Decreased levels |
|---|---|---|---|---|
| Parathyroid Hormone | See range published by individual laboratory | Slight ↑ | Primary or secondary hyperparathyoidism ↓ renal function with phosphate retention &/or low serum calcium Ectopic PTH prod (by tumors | High serum calcium |
| Calcitonin | See range published by individual laboratory | Slight ↓ | High serum calcium | Low serum calcium |
| Estrogen | M: 40–115 pg/mL F: 60–400 pg/mL (early menstrual cycle) 120–440 pg/mL (mid cycle) 150–350 pg/mL (late cycle) | M: gradual ↑ F: marked ↓ (<30 pg/mL in post-menopausal woman) | Ovarian tumor Adrenocortical tumor or hyperplasia Some testicular tumors | Ovarian failure Pituitary insufficiency Psychogenic stress |
| Luteinizing Hormone (LH) | M: 5–20 mIU/mL F: 5–25 mIU/mL (early in cycle) 40–80 mIU/mL (mid cycle) 5–25 mIU/mL (late cycle) | F: > 75 (postmenopausal) | Ovarian failure | Hypothalamic or pituitary hypofunction Testicular tumors Testicular failure |

218

| | | | | |
|---|---|---|---|---|
| Folicle Stimulating Hormone (FSH) | M: 10–15 mIU/mL<br>F: 5–25 mIU/mL (early in cycle)<br>20–30 mIU/mL (mid cycle)<br>5–25 mIU/mL (late cycle) | F: 40–250 (postmeno-pausal) | Ovarian failure | Hypothalamic or pituitary hypofunction<br>Testicular tumors |
| Prolactin | M: 1–20 ng/mL<br>F: 1–25 ng/mL | Progressive ↑ in males<br>F: 1–20 ng/mL | Any agent that depletes or antagonizes dopamine | Primary hypothyroidism<br>Pituitary adenomas<br>Lung or kidney tumors<br>↑ estrogen levels |
| Testosterone | M: 3.9–7.9 ng/mL<br>F: 0.25–0.67 ng/mL | M: Gradual ↓ until 7th decade when marked ↓ occurs<br>F: Slight ↓ to 0.21–0.37 ng/mL | Testicular tumors | Hypopituitarism<br>Testicular failure |

*Standard reference ranges cited from *Handbook of Laboratory and Diagnostic Tests With Nursing Implications* by J. L. Kee, (1990), Norwalk, CT: Appleton & Lange; and *Clinical Interpretation of Laboratory Tests* (9th ed) by F. K. Widmann, (1983), Philadelphia: F.A. Davis.

+The deviations listed are not an all-inclusive list, but are examples of deviations which may be seen in the elderly.

marrow cellularity from younger adult levels. Anemia is common in the elderly, but it is not caused by the aging process. By standard criteria, 21% of elderly women and 34% of elderly men have been reported to be anemic (Gambert, 1987, pp. 207–208).

The hemoglobin concentration decreases in both sexes after 65 years of age, particularly in men, due to reduced androgen production. Yet, while hemoglobin levels are normally higher in young adult males than females, the hemoglobin concentrations in the elderly of both sexes are nearly the same (Andres et al., 1985). Although women maintain their hematocrit levels throughout life, hematocrit values in men have been shown to decrease with age (Dever & Rothkopf, 1990, p. 104). In regard to other RBC indices, there is a slight increase in the mean corpuscular volume (MCV) with aging with no change in the mean corpuscular hemoglobin concentration (MCHC), since the cellular hemoglobin concentration rises proportionally (Gambert, 1987, p. 208).

The erythrocyte sedimentation rate (ESR) is reported by some authors (Gallo, Reichel, & Andersen, 1988, p. 162; Dever & Rothkopf, 1990, p. 104) as being slightly elevated in old age and somewhat higher in women. According to Gallo, Reichel, and Andersen, (1988, p. 162) the upper limit of normal for men <50 years of age is 15 mm/hr, while it is 20 mm/hr for men >50. They report the corresponding values for women to be 20 mm/hr and 30 mm/hr respectively. Conversely, Coodley (1990, p. 1186) contends that there is strong research evidence that age per se has no influence on the ESR. In this view, any age-related changes in ESR are best explained by the presence of a clinical disorder, such as an inflammatory process, a monoclonal gammopathy (an indicator of immune system dysregulation due to aging) or an elevated plasma fibrinogen level in association with a decrease in plasma albumin (Brocklehurst, 1985; Coodley, 1990, p. 1186).

## White Blood Cells

Although the total number of circulating white blood cells does not change significantly with age, white blood cell (WBC) function and production are less effective. This results in increased susceptibility to infections in older persons. In addition, signs and symptoms usually associated with leukocyte abnormalities may be different in the elderly; for example, signs of inflammation, fever, and lymph node enlargement may be reduced or absent in the presence of an acute infection (Andres et al., 1985).

A recent review of the literature revealed conflicting data concerning neutrophil counts of aged men and women (Rochman, 1988). This inconsistency makes the issue of whether there are age-related changes unclear. Although the neutrophil count does not appear to change with aging, there is research evidence that the rate of neutrophil release from the bone marrow may be reduced and that fewer of these cells are stored in the bone marrow (Andres et al., 1985). In addition, when older adults develop acute infections, immature forms of granulocytes are released from the bone marrow as in young adulthood, but without a significant increase in the absolute WBC count.

There does not appear to be an age-related change in the total lymphocyte count, but studies have consistently shown an age-related increase in the number of B cells (with a decline in B cell function) and no significant change in T cell number (but a significant decline in T cell function) (Lokhorst, Linden, Vander Schurman et al., 1983; Thompson, Wekstein, Rhoades et al., 1984; Wedelin, Bjorkholm, Holm et al., 1982). In regard to humoral immunity, antibody production in response to a specific stimulus is decreased while there is a paradoxical increase in autoantibody production (for example, causing low titers of anti-parietal cell, anti-mitochondrial, anti-thyroglobulin, anti-DNA antibody, and rheumatoid fever), in most cases without clinical symptoms. The decline in T cell function is related to a decrease in the differentiation of immature T cells by the atrophied thymus. This leads to a decline in cellular immunity with a poor T cell (hypersensitivity) response to new antigens (Gambert, 1987, p. 234).

Monocytes are similar to neutrophils in the way they perform to fight infection; however, unlike neutrophils, they have the capacity to become long-lived cells; thus, studies have shown that there is an increase in monocytes in both sexes with aging (Rochman, 1988). Although changes in *eosinophil* and *basophil* counts may occur in hypersensitivity reactions or parasitic infections, there is no evidence of age-related changes in these leukocytes (Rochman, 1988).

## Platelets

There is no significant change in the platelet count associated with normal aging (Rock, 1984, p. 58). In addition, there is no change in prothrombin time (PT) and partial thromboplastin time (PTT) in healthy elders. There is no conclusive evidence that clotting increases, but there is some evidence that fibrinogen levels increase with age (Garner, 1989, p. 144).

## BLOOD GASES

Arterial pH and $PaCO_2$ are unchanged with normal aging. However, there is a gradual decrease in arterial $PaO_2$. In addition, both the central and peripheral respiratory drive in older individuals decline in response to any increase in the $PaCO_2$ and decrease in the $PaO_2$ (Gambert, 1987, p. 51).

## BLOOD CHEMISTRIES

Although the reported data are not entirely consistent, the ranges of most biochemical test results in the elderly are, with few exceptions, not very different from those in younger adults (Coodley, 1990, p. 1185).

### Serum Iron and Ferritin

In association with other evidence of defective iron utilization, such as increased marrow iron and serum ferritin (reflecting stored iron), there is a progressive decrease in serum iron levels with age in both men and women. In the 71 to 80 year age group, the serum iron level is 50 to 75% of the serum iron levels of young adults; in younger adults it ranges from 115 to 130 ug/dl, compared to 70 to 80 ug/dl in old age (Gambert, 1987, p. 209). A low serum ferritin concentration is a more sensitive indicator of iron deficiency (Gallo et al., 1988, p. 161).

It is important to distinguish between age-related decreases of serum iron and/or serum ferritin and anemia. Anemia is not a normal consequence of aging and may be caused by dietary deficiencies and a number of disease states. Poor appetite, inadequate consumption of iron-rich foods, poor iron absorption, and/or chronic blood loss— especially from the GI track—may place the older person at risk for developing iron-deficiency anemia. However, it should be remembered in the differential diagnosis of anemia that elderly individuals may develop any of the other types of anemia as well.

### Vitamin $B_{12}$

With advancing age there is a moderate decrease in serum $B_{12}$ levels, possibly due to decreased intrinsic factor secretion with impaired $B_{12}$ absorption (Dever & Rothkopf, 1990, p. 105). By the 7th decade, vitamin $B_{12}$ levels are from 60% to 80% of those in young adults (Dykbauer, Lauritzan, & Krakauer, 1981). Although serum $B_{12}$ levels below 100 mg/dl definitely indicate a deficiency, levels between 100 and 200 mg/dl are indeterminate, especially in the absence of macrocytosis (Gambert, 1987, p. 218). Although there is a direct relationship between poor nutrition and low vitamin $B_{12}$ levels (Roe, 1983), an age-related decline in vitamin $B_{12}$ values has been documented in healthy populations of young and old with comparable dietary intake (Garry et al.,

1983). It is important to differentiate vitamin B$_{12}$ deficiency from the moderate age-related decline in this laboratory value, because neurologic deficits and/or dementia may develop prior to the onset of anemia symptoms and become irreversible if not promptly treated. As at any age, the Shilling test is required to identify the cause of a vitamin B$_{12}$ deficiency (Gambert, 1987, p. 218).

## Folic Acid

No age-related changes in the serum level of folic acid have been documented; however, measurement of erythrocyte (RBC) folate is a more reliable test for determining true folate deficiency. A decrease in this laboratory value should prompt a search for dietary insufficiency (the most common cause), tropical sprue, or inflammatory bowel disease, or ingestion of antifolic agents such as alcohol, anticonvulsants, or sulfa drugs (Dever & Rothkopf, 1990, p. 105).

## Glucose

Pancreatic insulin supply declines and its release is slower with age. Factors that contribute to changes in glucose metabolism and increasing blood glucose values with aging include a decrease in lean body mass without a significant change in total body weight (that is, increased adiposity). As a result of decline in lean body mass, less tissue is available for glucose uptake. Decreased physical activity is also associated with a decrease in insulin sensitivity. The presence of the classic triad of symptoms (polyuria, polydipsia, and polyphagia) and an elevated blood sugar value, plus weight loss with glycosuria and ketonuria, is usually sufficient for the diagnosis of insulin dependent diabetes mellitus (IDDM) in an older adult. However, it is especially difficult to determine whether increasing glucose values in older individuals without these other signs and symptoms are the result of the aging process or noninsulin dependent diabetes mellitus (NIDDM) (Andres et al., 1985; Brocklehurst, 1985).

The fasting blood glucose (FBG) rises at a rate of approximately 2 mg/dl per decade after 35 (Gallo et al., 1988, p. 164). Starting in the 3rd decade, the 1 hour plasma glucose following oral glucose ingestion also gradually increases between 4 to 14 mg/dl per decade (mean = 9 mg/dl) and the 2 hour plasma glucose increases from 1 to 11 mg/dl per decade (mean = 5 mg/dl). The mean 1 hour plasma glucose is 100 mg/dl at age 18 to 24, and rises to 166 mg/dl by age 75 to 79. The National Diabetes Data Group criteria for diagnosing diabetes in the elderly include: fasting plasma glucose equal to or greater than 140 mg/dl on more than one occasion; or plasma glucose 2 hours following ingestion of 1.75 g/kg (up to 75 g) glucose exceeding 200 mg/dl *and* at least one other glucose value during the 2-hour oral glucose tolerance test exceeding 200 mg/dl (Gambert, 1987, pp. 166–167).

## Cholesterol

As a result of changes in lipid metabolism with advancing age, total cholesterol levels, as well as triglyceride levels, have been reported to gradually increase with age in both sexes. Although younger women have lower total cholesterol levels than younger men, this sex-related difference decreases significantly in the elderly (Rock, 1984, p. 60). A fasting lipid profile which reports the HDL ("good" cholesterol) and LDL ("bad" cholesterol) fractions and their ratio are the best indicators of risk for coronary disease in the elderly as in younger age groups. Women tend to have higher $HDL_2$ subfractions than men throughout life. While increases in HDL cholesterol in women have been documented between the 3rd and 7th decades, these levels decrease in men after the first decade of life until the 7th decade when slight increases may be noted. Although little is presently known about the benefits of treatment of borderline elevations of LDL-cholesterol in the healthy older person, lifestyle modifications, such as moderate fat restriction, increased fiber intake, and exercise can be encouraged for their overall health benefits. As at earlier ages, a significant increase in LDL-cholesterol in conjunction with a decreased HDL-cholesterol warrants aggressive treatment (Gambert, 1987, pp. 177–179).

## Serum Proteins

There is no change in total serum proteins with aging. Studies have not documented a significant decrease in serum albumin in healthy older persons. Average values decline less than 0.5g/ml with age; this change is balanced by a slight increase in B globulin (Garner, 1989, p. 144). The decrease in serum albumin that is found in some elderly, especially those who are hospitalized, may be more related to diet than to the aging process (Coodley, 1990, p. 1186).

## Blood Urea Nitrogen and Serum Creatinine

Due to age-related changes in kidney function, the blood urea nitrogen (BUN) tends to increase with age in both men and women, although average values in females are lower than those of males (Hale, Stewart, & Marks, 1983). Many factors other than kidney function can affect the BUN value, including fluid and protein intake, liver function, and GI bleeding. The BUN/creatinine ratio can provide an estimate of the specific contribution of renal function to an elevated BUN value. The normal ratio is 10:1 and, if the BUN is raised out of proportion to the creatinine level (for example, the ratio is 15 or 20:1), there may be underlying renal disease (Gallo et al., 1988, p. 163).

Despite a 0.6%/year decline in renal function after reaching maturity, serum creatinine varies little with age. This is because a concomitant decrease in muscle mass results in a decrease in endogenous creatinine formation (Gambert, 1987, p. 121). Therefore, even in early renal failure, the serum creatinine may remain within the limits of normal. In addition, when renal function is changing rapidly, the creatinine may remain within the limits of normal, and does not accurately reflect the glomerular filtration rate (GFR) or creatinine clearance at any given moment (Gallo et al., 1988, p. 162). Although the 24-hour urine creatinine clearance test shows a progressive decline with age (Rossman, 1986), it is a more accurate indicator of glomerular dysfunction in the elderly at any given moment than the serum creatinine alone. However, glomerular function can be estimated on a timed 8-hour urine collection (e.g., overnight). Alternatively, when only the serum creatinine is available, the influence of age can be estimated by the following formula:

$$\text{Creatinine clearance} = \frac{(140 - \text{age}) \times \text{body wt (kg)}}{72 \times \text{serum creatinine (mg/dl)}}$$

For women, multiply by 0.85 (Abrams & Berkow, 1990, p. 188). Further research is needed to develop more precise estimates of the relationship between age, weight, serum creatinine, and creatinine clearance for the older population (Drusano, Muncie, Hoopes et al., 1988).

## Uric Acid

There is an age-related increase in serum uric acid levels, particularly in women. This change occurs during the 4th or 5th decade and is related to perimenopausal hormonal shifts. Men, at all ages, have higher uric acid levels than women, but have a less dramatic increase as they age (Rochman, 1988). Therefore, men have a higher risk of gout regardless of age, while the risk of gout in women increases after menopause.

## Serum Electrolytes

Although the elderly may be more susceptible to a variety of electrolyte imbalances because of factors such as medication side-effects and poor fluid intake, serum electrolytes are rarely abnormal because of age alone (Coodley, 1990, p. 1185). Potassium imbalance is the only electrolyte disturbance which has an age-frequency distribution. Serum potassium levels remain constant until the 6th decade, when a slight age-related increase occurs. Up to 30% of nursing home residents and other frail elderly may have abnormal potassium levels because of dietary insufficiency, continued use of diuretics or laxatives, or physiological alterations such as diarrhea or diabetic acidosis. It is important to recognize hyperkalemia in the elderly (which may result from renal failure, use of potassium-sparing diuretics or salt substitutes composed largely of potassium, adrenal insufficiency, acidosis, and/or hyponatremia) because it can cause serious cardiac and neuromuscular dysfunction. Early detection of hypokalemia (which can result from decreased intake, increased loss from the GI track or renal excretion, or endocrine disorders) is also important, since it is associated with cardiac arrhythmias, digitalis toxicity, and renal tubular dysfunction (Dever & Rothkopf, 1990, p. 109).

## Serum Enzyme Levels

Alkaline phosphatase gradually increases with age in both sexes, with the increase being more marked in women. The concomitant increase in another liver enzyme (GGT) suggests that this increase is hepatic rather than osseous in origin (Coodley, 1990, p. 1186). In healthy older adults the normal values may be up to 1 to 1½ times the standard normal value. Age- and sex-adjusted normal ranges should be used when interpreting the older person's creatine phosphokinase (CPK) values. While increased CPK values are usually seen with myocardial infarction (MI) in younger adults, total CPK values may not be abnormally elevated in older adults. When MI is suspected in an older client, CPK isoenzyme separation (CPK-MB) is necessary to confirm this diagnosis (Dever & Rothkopf, 1990, p. 107). The normal range for serum gamma glutamyl transpeptidase (GGT) for females over 45 years of age is slightly higher than for younger females; there is no age-related change in normal values of this liver enzyme for males (Morton, 1989). Laboratory values for lactate dehydrogenase (LDH), glutamic-pyruvic transaminase (SGPT), and glutamic-oxaloacetic transaminase (SGOT) do not significantly change during the normal aging process (Dever & Rothkopf, 1990, p. 107).

## ENDOCRINE STUDIES

Differentiation between the effects of normal age changes and endocrine disorders in older persons is challenging because the normal aging process is associated with alterations in hormone production, secretion, and biologic effect. In addition, normal age changes in the renal, pulmonary, gastrointestinal, and hepatic systems complicate endocrine test interpretation and diagnosis. The use of age-related endocrine test reference values is particularly important to facilitate the interpretation of laboratory results in older individuals with subtle manifestations of endocrine disease (Demers, 1988, p. 24).

## Thyroid Indices

The rate of production of thyroid hormone is estimated to decrease by 50% between 20 to 80 years of age (Brocklehurst, 1988). While many of the signs and symptoms of hypothyroidism (for example, weakness, lethargy, dry skin, poor memory, constipation, and cold intolerance) may mistakenly be attributed to the aging process, hyperthyroidism may manifest itself in the older person with very atypical signs and symptoms (for example, lethargy, apathetic facies, anorexia, depression, and cardiovascular abnormalities). In addition, interpretation of thyroid function tests is complicated by concurrent disease; ill elderly who are actually euthyroid may have a decreased $T_3$ or an elevated $T_4$ (Gallo et al., 1988, p. 163). Therefore, laboratory tests play an especially important role in the diagnosis of thyroid dysfunction in the elderly. It is important that reference values be based on older adult populations and that laboratory values be looked at within the context of the whole clinical picture. For example, if an older client with clinical signs and symptoms of hyperthyroidism has normal serum $T_4$ levels, measurement of serum $T_3$ is essential because autonomous thyroid nodules are more common in the elderly (Gambert, 1987, pp. 159–160).

There is a slight decrease in circulating thyroxine ($T_4$) with age (Demers, 1988) which may be caused by a decrease in the rate of metabolic processes and hormone production in the aging thyroid gland. Triiodothyro-nine ($T_3$), the active form of thyroid hormone (derived principally from peripheral deiodination of $T_4$), has also been shown to decrease from 10 to 50% in older populations due to decreased peripheral conversion of $T_4$ to $T_3$. This means that a $T_3$ level near the upper limit of normal may be the only abnormal thyroid hormone value associated with clinical signs of hyperthyroidism in an older individual, while a younger client with the same result would be asymptomatic (Gambert, 1987, p. 156). While male $T_3$ levels begin to decrease at age 60, females do not show a consistent decrease until age 70 to 80 (Rochman, 1988).

As the thyroid's ability to maintain a euthyroid state declines with aging, proportionally more $T_3$ than $T_4$ is produced (the ratio changes from 15:1 in youth, to 5:1 in later life). In addition, the half life of $T_4$ increases from 5 days in youth to over 9 days by the 9th decade

(Gambert, 1987, pp. 156–157). These normal changes in the $T_4$ and $T_3$ levels and their ratio make it more difficult to diagnose mild hypothyroidism or hyperthyroidism in the elderly and have profound implications for thyroid replacement therapy in this age group. The $T_3$ Resin Uptake test ($T_3RU$) is useful only in conjunction with other thyroid function tests, especially the free thyroxine index (FTI). Free hormone levels are the best indicators of thyroid function since many other factors (for example, numerous drugs and disease states, pregnancy, and stress) affect the $T_3RU$ and total serum thyroxine levels (Gambert, 1987, pp. 157–158).

Repeated studies have shown an age-related increase in serum thyroid-stimulating hormone (TSH) in both men and women over 60 years of age (Harman, Whemann, & Blackman, 1984; Rochman, 1988). This is because many older persons have a failing but compensated thyroid status. Therefore, a slightly elevated TSH may indicate a partially compensated thyroid gland or true hypothyroidism (if there is a concomitant decrease in serum $T_4$). The serum TSH is the most sensitive indicator of hypothyroidism. It is still controversial as to whether a slight TSH increase (when the serum $T_4$ and $T_3$ are normal) should be treated with hormone replacement (Gambert, 1987, p. 163). However, elders with elevated antimicrosomal antibodies are definitely more likely to develop clinically overt hypothyroidism and may require prophylactic hormone replacement therapy (Gallo et al., 1988, p. 163).

This age-related increase in TSH must also be considered when interpreting the results of the thyrotropin-releasing hormone (TRH) stimulation test. Studies have shown that there is a decrease in the expected surge of TSH secretion by the pituitary in response to administration of TRH in healthy older men (Rochman, 1988). Therefore, this should not be automatically considered to indicate a thyroid disorder.

## Other Hormone Levels

The progressive increase in prolactin in aging men may be related to a gradual increase in serum estrogen. Increased serum and urinary estrogen in older men are derived from androstenedione, which is metabolized to estrogen by peripheral tissues. An increase in the serum level of luteinizing hormone (LH), and an even greater increase in the follicle stimulating hormone (FSH) serum level begins during the 5th decade in men; but these changes are much more pronounced in postmenopausal women (Coodley, 1990, p. 1187).

The decrease in serum testosterone levels in the elderly may be due entirely to aging, or may be influenced by environmental factors such as stress, minor illnesses, or decreased physical activity. Free testosterone levels, in general, are less affected by age than morning levels and the mean 24-hour plasma testosterone. A marked decrease in serum testosterone does not occur until after the 7th decade. Increased gonadotrophin levels in older men may be the result of decreased testosterone secretion. In general, serum renin, endorphins, and calcitonin decrease slightly with aging, while parathyroid hormone levels increase with age (Coodley, 1990, p. 1187).

## NURSING IMPLICATIONS

Nurses frequently note and interpret laboratory values in their practice, synthesizing this data with information from the health history and physical, psychosocial, and functional assessments in developing appropriate nursing care plans for older clients. The older person's changing laboratory values reflect normal aging, as well as disease states and the effects of medical therapies. This makes valid interpretation of the changing laboratory values of older individuals a challenging task.

While research with healthy populations of older people to date indicates that the normal ranges for many test results do not change as a result of the aging process, changes in the range of normal values for a number of other laboratory tests do need to be considered in assessing the health status of older clients. It is important for the practitioner to evaluate the laboratory test results of older persons within the context of normal age changes, as well as with consideration of the possibility of altered presentations of many illnesses and the possibility of iatrogenesis.

Recognition of age-related variations from the norms of younger adults can prevent overtreatment of conditions such as mild hyperglycemia in the elderly. In addition, knowledge concerning the laboratory values that remain unchanged during normal aging can help the care provider to recognize laboratory results that are abnormal in older as well as younger adults and to see that causative conditions such as anemia are adequately treated, rather than mistakenly being attributed to aging and, therefore, ignored.

## REFERENCES

Abrams, W. B., & Berkow, R. (Eds.). (1990). *The Merck manual of geriatrics.* Rahway, NJ: Merck, Sharp, & Dohne.

Andres, R., Bierman, E., & Hazzard, W. (1985). *Principles of geriatric medicine.* New York: McGraw-Hill.

Brocklehurst, J. (1985). *Textbook of geriatric medicine and gerontology* (3rd ed). New York: Churchill Livingstone.

Burrage, R. L., Dixon, L., & Sehy, Y. A. (1991). Physical Assessment: An Overview. In Chenitz, W. C., Stone, J. T., & Salisbury, S. A. (Eds.), *Clinical gerontological nursing: A guide to advanced practice* (p. 32). Philadelphia: W. B. Saunders.

Demers, L. (1988). The aging endocrine system. *Lab Management, 26,* 24.

Dever, A. M., & Rothkopf, R. M. (1990). Laboratory values and implications in care of the aged. In Ebersole, P., & Hess, P. (Eds.), *Toward healthy aging: Human needs and nursing responses* (pp. 101–109). St. Louis: C.V. Mosby.

Drusano, G., Muncie, H., Hoopes, J., et al. (1988). Commonly used methods of estimating creatinine clearance are inadequate for elderly debilitated nursing home patients. *Journal of the American Geriatrics Society, 36,* 437.

Dykbauer, R., Lauritzen, M., & Krakauer, R. (1981). Relative reference values for clinical chemical and haematological quantities in "healthy" elderly people. *Acta Medica Scandinavica, 209,* 1.

Coodley, E. (1990). Changes in laboratory values. In Abrams, W. B., & Berkow, R. (Eds.), *The Merck manual of geriatrics* (pp. 1185–1187). Rahway, NJ: Merck Sharp & Dohme Research Laboratories.

Gallo, J. J., Reichel, W., & Andersen, L. (1988). *Handbook of geriatric assessment* (pp. 161–164). Gaithersburg, MD: Aspen Publishers, Inc.

Gambert, S. R. (Ed.). (1987). *Handbook of geriatrics.* New York: Plenum Medical Book Co.

Garner, B. C. (1989). Guide to changing lab values in elders. *Geriatric Nursing, 10*(3), 144.

Garry, P.J . et al. (1983). Iron status and anemia in the elderly: New findings and a review of previous studies. *Journal of the American Geriatrics Society, 31,* 389–399.

Hale, W., Stewart, R., & Marks, R. (1983). Haematological and biochemical laboratory values in an ambulatory elderly population: An analysis of the effects of age, sex, and drugs. *Age Aging, 12,* 275.

Harman, S., Whemann, R., & Blackman, M. (1984). Pituitary-thyroid hormone economy in healthy aging men: Basal indices of thyroid function and thyrotropin responses to constant infusions of thyrotrotropin releasing hormone. *Journal of Clinical Endocrinology and Metabolism, 23,* 101.

Kane, R. L., Ouslander, J. G., & Abrass, I. B. (1989). *Essentials of clinical geriatrics* (2nd ed) (p. 61). New York: McGraw Hill.

Lokhorst, H., Linden, J., Vander Schurman, H. et al. (1983). Immune function during aging in man: Relation between serological abnormalities and cellular immune status. *European Journal of Clinical Investigation, 13,* 209.

Morton, P. G. (1989). *Health assessment in nursing* (p. 381). Springhouse, PA: Springhouse Corp.

Rochman, H. (1988). *Clinical pathology in the elderly.* New York: Karger.

Rock, R. C. (1984). Effects of age on common laboratory tests. *Geriatrics, 39*(6), 57–60.

Roe, D. (1983). *Geriatric nutrition*. Englewood Cliffs, NJ: Prentice-Hall.

Rossman, I. (1986). *Clinical geriatrics* (3rd ed). Philadelphia: J.B. Lippincott.

Thompson, J., Wekstein, D., Rhoades, J. et al. (1984). The immune status of healthy centenarians. *Journal of the American Geriatrics Society, 32*, 274.

Wedelin, C., Bjorkholm, M., Holm, G. et al. (1982). Blood T-lymphocyte function in healthy adults in relation to age. *Scandinavian Journal of Haematology, 28*, 45.

## SUGGESTED READINGS

Brocklehurst, J. (1985). *Textbook of geriatric medicine and gerontology* (3rd ed). New York: Churchill Livingstone.

Chenitz, W. C., Stone, J. T., & Salisbury, S. A. (Eds.). (1991). *Clinical gerontological nursing: A guide to advanced practice*. Philadelphia: W.B. Saunders.

Ebersole, P., & Hess, P. (Eds.). (1990). *Towards health aging: Human needs and human responses*. St. Louis: C.V. Mosby.

Friedman, R. B., & Young, D. S. (1989). *Effects of disease on clinical laboratory tests*. Washington, DC: AACC Press.

Gallo, J. J., Reichel, W., & Andersen, L. (1988). *Handbook of geriatric assessment*. Gaithersburg, MD: Aspen Publishers, Inc.

Gambert, S. R. (Ed.). (1987). *Handbook of geriatrics*. New York: Plenum Medical Book Co.

Garner, B. C. (1989). Guide to changing lab values in eldero. *Geriatric Nursing, 10*(3), 144–145.

Kane, R. L., Ouslander, J. G., & Abrass, I. B. (1989). *Essentials of clinical geriatrics* (2nd ed). New York: McGraw Hill.

Kee, J. L. (1990). *Handbook of laboratory and diagnostic tests with nursing implications*. Norwalk, CT: Appleton & Lange.

Morton, P. G. (1989). *Health assessment in nursing*. Springhouse, PA: Springhouse Corp.

Roberts, G. H., & Ramsey, M. K. (1990). Interpretive clinical chemistry laboratory tests. *Journal of Pharmacy Technology, 6*, 21–28.

Rock, R. C. (1984). Effects of age on common laboratory tests. *Geriatrics, 39*(6), 57–60.

Rossman, I. (1986). *Clinical geriatrics* (3rd ed). Philadelphia: J.B. Lippincott.

Tietz, N. W. (1987). *Fundamentals of clinical chemistry*. Philadelphia: W. B. Saunders.

Tilkian, S. M., Conover, M. B., & Tilkian, A. G. (1987). *Clinical implications of laboratory tests*. St. Louis: C.V. Mosby.

Widmann, F. K. (1983). *Clinical interpretation of laboratory tests* (9th ed). Philadelphia: F.A. Davis Company.

# Appendix

---

## KEY HEALTH STATUS OBJECTIVES TARGETING OLDER ADULTS

Reduce suicides among white men aged 65 and older to no more than 39.2 per 100,000. (Age-adjusted baseline: 46.1 per 100,000 in 1987)

Reduce deaths among people aged 70 and older caused by motor vehicle crashes to no more than 20 per 100,000. (Baseline: 22.6 per 100,000 in 1987)

Reduce deaths among people aged 65 through 84 from falls and fall-related injuries to no more than 14.4 per 100,000. (Baseline: 18 per 100,000 in 1987)

Reduce deaths among people aged 85 and older from falls and fall-related injuries to no more than 105 per 100,000. (Baseline 131.2 per 100,000 in 1987)

Reduce residential fire deaths among people aged 65 and older to no more than 3.3 per 100,000. (Baseline: 4.4 per 100,000 in 1987)

Reduce hip fractures among people aged 65 and older so that hospitalizations for this condition are no more than 607 per 100,000. (Baseline: 714 per 100,000 in 1988)

|  | Special Population Target | |
|---|---|---|
| *Hip Fractures* (per 100,000) | *1988 Baseline* | *2000 Target* |
| White women aged 85 and older | 2,721 | 2,177 |

Reduce to no more than 20 percent the proportion of people aged 65 and older who have lost all of their natural teeth. (Baseline: 36 percent in 1986)

*Special Population Target*

| Complete Tooth Loss Prevalence | 1986 Baseline | 2000 Target |
|---|---|---|
| Low-income people (annual family income <$15,000) | 46% | 25% |

Increase years of healthy life to at least 65 years. (Baseline: An estimated 62 years in 1980)

*Special Population Targets*

| Years of Healthy Life | 1980 Baseline | 2000 Target |
|---|---|---|
| Blacks | 56 | 60 |
| Hispanics | 62 | 65 |
| People aged 65 and older | 12† | 14† |

†*Years of healthy life remaining at age 65*

*Note: Years of healthy life (also referred to as quality-adjusted life years) is a summary measure of health that combines mortality (quantity of life) and morbidity and disability (quality of life) into a single measure. For people aged 65 and older, active life-expectancy, a related summary measure, also will be tracked.*

Reduce to no more than 90 per 1,000 people the proportion of all people aged 65 and older who have difficulty in performing two or more personal care activities, thereby preserving independence. (Baseline: 111 per 1,000 in 1984–85)

*Special Population Target*

| Difficulty Performing Self-Care Activities (per 1,000) | 1984–85 Baseline | 2000 Target |
|---|---|---|
| People aged 85 and older | 371 | 325 |

*Note: Personal care activities are bathing, dressing, using the toilet, getting in and out of bed or chair, and eating.*

Reduce significant hearing impairment among people aged 45 and older to a prevalence of no more than 180 per 1,000. (Baseline: Average of 203 per 1,000 during 1986–88)

*Note: Hearing impairment covers the range of hearing deficits from mild loss in one ear to profound loss in both ears. Generally, inability to hear sounds at levels softer (less intense) than 20 decibels (dB) constitutes abnormal hearing. Significant hearing impairment is defined as having hearing thresholds for speech poorer than 25 dB. However, for this objective, self-reported hearing impairment (i.e., deafness in one or both ears or any trouble hearing in one or both ears) will be used as a proxy measure for significant hearing impairment.*

Reduce significant visual impairment among people aged 65 and older to a prevalence of no more than 70 per 1,000. (Baseline: Average of 87.1 per 1,000 during 1986–88)

*Note: Significant visual impairment is generally defined as a permanent reduction in visual acuity and/or field of vision which is not correctable with eyeglasses or contact lenses. Severe visual impairment is defined as inability to read ordinary newsprint even with corrective lenses.*

*For this objective, self-reported blindness in one or both eyes and other self-reported visual impairments (e.g., any trouble seeing with one or both eyes even when wearing glasses or colorblindness) will be used as a proxy measure for significant visual impairment.*

Reduce epidemic-related pneumonia and influenza deaths among people aged 65 and older to no more than 7.3 per 100,000. (Baseline: Average of 9.1 per 100,000 during 1980 through 1987)

*Epidemic-related pneumonia and influenza deaths are those that occur above and beyond the normal yearly fluctuations of mortality. Because of the extreme variability in epidemic-related deaths from year to year, the target is a 3-year average.*

Reduce pneumonia-related days of restricted activity as follows:

|                                                | 1987 Baseline | 2000 Target |
|------------------------------------------------|---------------|-------------|
| People aged 65 and older (per 100 people)      | 48 days       | 38 days     |

## KEY RISK REDUCTION OBJECTIVES TARGETING OLDER ADULTS

Reduce to no more than 22 percent the proportion of people aged 65 and older who engage in no leisure-time physical activity. (Baseline: 43 percent in 1985)

*Note: For this objective, people with disabilities are people who report any limitation in activity due to chronic conditions.*

Increase immunization levels as follows:

Pneumococcal pneumonia and influenza immunization among institutionalized chronically ill or older people: at least 80 percent. (Baseline data available in 1992)

Increase to at least 40 percent the proportion of adults aged 65 and older who have received, as a minimum within the appropriate interval, all of the screening and immunization services and at least one of the counseling services appropriate for their age and gender as recommended by the U.S. Preventive Services Task Force. (Baseline data available in 1991)

## KEY SERVICES AND PROTECTION OBJECTIVES TARGETING OLDER ADULTS

Increase to at least 80 percent the receipt of home food services by people aged 65 and older who have difficulty in preparing their own meals or are otherwise in need of home-delivered meals. (Baseline data available in 1991)

Increase to at least 90 percent the proportion of people aged 65 and older who had the opportunity to participate during the preceding year in at least one organized health promotion program through a senior center, lifecare facility, or other community-based setting that serves older adults. (Baseline data available in 1992)

Increase to at least 30 the number of States that have design standards for signs, signals, markings, lighting, and other characteristics of the roadway environment to improve the visual stimuli and protect the safety of older drivers and pedestrians. (Baseline data available in 1992)

Increase to at least 75 percent the proportion of primary care providers who routinely review with their patients aged 65 and older all prescribed and over-the-counter medicines taken by their patients each time a new medication is prescribed. (Baseline data available in 1992)

Extend to all long-term institutional facilities the requirement that oral examinations and services be provided no later than 90 days after entry into these facilities. (Baseline: Nursing facilities receiving Medicaid or Medicare reimbursement will be required to provide for oral examinations within 90 days of patient entry beginning in 1990; baseline data unavailable for other institutions)

*Note: Long-term institutional facilities include nursing homes, prisons, juvenile homes, and detention facilities.*

Increase to at least 60 percent the proportion of people aged 65 and older using the oral health care system during each year. (Baseline: 42 percent in 1986)

Increase to at least 80 percent the proportion of women aged 40 and older who have ever received a clinical breast examination and a mammogram, and to at least 60 percent those aged 50 and older who have received them within the preceding 1 to 2 years. (Baseline: 36 percent of women aged 40 and older "ever" in 1987; 25 percent of women aged 50 and older "within the preceding 2 years" in 1987)

*Special Population Targets*

| Clinical Breast Exam & Mammogram Ever Received— | 1987 Baseline | 2000 Target |
|---|---|---|
| Hispanic women aged 40 and older | 20% | 80% |
| Low-income women aged 40 and older (annual family income <$10,000) | 22% | 80% |
| Women aged 40 and older with less than high school education | 23% | 80% |
| Women aged 70 and older | 25% | 80% |
| Black women aged 40 and older | 28% | 80% |

*Received Within Preceding 2 Years—*

| | | |
|---|---|---|
| Hispanic women aged 50 and older | 18% | 60% |
| Low-income women aged 50 and older (annual family income <$10,000) | 15% | 60% |
| Women aged 50 and older with less than high school education | 16% | 60% |
| Women aged 70 and older | 18% | 60% |
| Black women aged 50 and older | 19% | 60% |

Increase to at least 95 percent the proportion of women aged 70 and older with uterine cervix who have ever received a Pap test, and to at least 70 percent those who received a Pap test within the preceding 1 to 3 years. (Baseline: 76 percent "ever" and 44 percent "within the preceding 3 years" in 1987)

Increase to at least 50 percent the proportion of people aged 50 and older who have received fecal occult blood testing within the preceding 1 to 2 years, and to at least 40 percent those who have ever received proctosigmoidoscopy. (Baseline: 27 percent received fecal occult blood testing during the preceding 2 years in 1987; 25 percent had ever received proctosigmoidoscopy in 1987)

Increase to at least 40 percent the proportion of people aged 50 and older visiting a primary care provider in the preceding year who have received oral, skin, and digital rectal examinations during one such visit. (Baseline: An estimated 27 percent received a digital rectal exam during a physician visit within the preceding year in 1987)

Increase to at least 60 percent the proportion of providers of primary care for older adults who routinely evaluate people aged 65 and older for urinary incontinence and impairments of vision, hearing, cognition, and functional status. (Baseline data available in 1992)

Increase to at least 90 percent the proportion of perimenopausal women who have been counseled about the benefits and risks of estrogen replacement therapy (combined with progestin, when appropriate) for prevention of osteoporosis. (Baseline data available in 1991)

Except as otherwise noted, all rates in the following objectives are annual. Where the baseline rate is age adjusted, it is age adjusted to the 1940 U.S. population, and the target is age adjusted also.

*Note*: U.S. Department of Health and Human Services. *Healthy People 2000: National Health Promotion and Disease Prevention* (1991). Rockville, MD: Public Health Service.

# Index